D1435201

OEDIPUS ROAD

OEDIPUS ROAD

Searching for a Father in a Mother's Fading Memory

TOM DODGE

ASBURY PARK PUBLIC LIBRARY
ASBURY PARK, NEW JERSEY

Texas Christian University Press / Fort Worth

Copyright © 1996, Tom Dodge

Library of Congress Cataloging-in-Publication Data

Dodge, Tom, 1939-
   Oedipus Road : searching for a father in a mother's fading memory / by Tom Dodge
   p. cm.
   ISBN 0-87565-153-4
   1. Mothers and sons—United States—Case studies. 2. Parent and adult child—United States—Case studies. 3. Paternal deprivation—United States—Case studies. 4. Alzeheimer's disease—Patients—United States—Family relationships. 5. Caregivers—United States—Case studies. I. Title.

   HQ755.85. D64 1996
   306.874'3—dc20

                                               95-26697
                                               CIP

Portions of this book have been used in Tom Dodge's commentaries on radio station KERA, Dallas, Texas.

Text and cover design by Barbara Whitehead

To my Aunt Bernice Patterson

And then when they had passed beyond the throne of Necessity, they journeyed together to the Plain of Lethe. When evening came, they encamped beside the River of Forgetfulness, whose water no vessel can hold. All are required to drink a certain measure of this water, and some have not the wisdom to save them from drinking more. All who drink forget everything. When they had fallen asleep, there was thunder and an earthquake, and in a moment they were carried up, this way and that, to their birth, like shooting stars.... And so ... all will be well when we cross the River of Lethe.

Plato, *The Republic*

FOREWORD

On Mother's Day of 1994 I took my mother to her favorite theme park, Wal-Mart, and bought her a few gifts that she selected. If she doesn't pick them out, she throws them out. Our children brought her cards. We talked for a long time about her new items and the cards. She smiled and looked at each of them lovingly. She's amazingly youthful looking at seventy-six—slender without a noticeable gray hair, and she still laughs often and easily. Her love of the absurd is intact: a fat man, his pants hanging low, devouring a barbecued chicken leg, can send her into fits of cackling delight. It is a spontaneous, bright and joyous laugh, one that endears her to grown-ups and children alike. She has always been playful, a talented mimic, childlike herself and boundlessly accommodating to other children:

"Juanita, that child is wrapping her tea dishes with the pages from your hundred-year-old family Bible!"

"Bless her little angel heart. We can get another one."

This kind of thing.

Her expertise with children is legendary among members of the First Baptist Church in Cleburne, where she worked in the nursery for twenty-five years. When she finally, mercifully, retired in 1992, the church responded with an appreciation ceremony during Sunday services. When the pastor asked members to stand who had either been under her care or whose children had, three-fourths of the congregation stood up. Her co-workers gave her several gifts and a plaque, and the pastor delivered a warm tribute, glowing with encomiums. Parents, he said, soon learned that their children didn't want to go home with them after staying in the nursery with Juanita. Then he asked her if she had anything she wanted to say. "Keep going," she said, "you're doing fine."

With children, myself included, my mother seemed to have the golden touch. Growing up, I could count on her for money to buy movie tickets, comic books, ball gloves, and the like. She took me to softball games, to movies, to carnivals when they came to town, and to the zoo once. Throughout my life, including the thirteen years that we lived together in the same household, she was never abusive in any way or even critical.

I wish we had gotten to know one another better.

I thought that her first Mother's Day in Midlothian had come and gone without incident. She was settled into the house across the street from us—so close that I could see it easily from my kitchen window—and now night was falling and all was well. Brenda, my wife, just home from a trip, had hardly had time to put her bags down, and I was standing by the sink thinking how great life was now that I had finally solved my "mother problem." I was contemplating the joys of freedom—making a list of all the things I would do with my extra time now that I didn't have to make the daily trip of twenty-five miles to Cleburne to see after her. This foolish revery was interrupted when my mother suddenly appeared in our kitchen. My eyes saw that she was carrying something in her hand, but my brain said, "He doesn't want to know what that item is" and refused to translate the information. But even the most protective of brains can stonewall only so long. "My god," I thought, "my mother's got a condom in her hand!"

The pernicious prophylactic was fully extended, and she was waving it around like an airport windsock. She held it out and said, "Look what I found in my driveway. Why would anybody do this to me?" Then, she under-handed the reprehensible rubber onto our dining room table. It came to rest in the fruit bowl and dangled off the side of a fresh pineapple.

I reacted just exactly as my brain knew I would. "What is wrong with you?" I yelled. (This was an extremely fool-ish thing to say because I knew exactly what was wrong with her.) "Bring a condom in my house and pitch it on the dining room table? On Mother's Day?" It was a big dramatic outburst. About five seconds into this over-wrought exhibition, I remembered that I was supposed to be the rational one.

What I should have said was: "That's nice, Mom. Now, would you like some coffee?"

After cooling down I explained to her that, although I'm not exactly the most sentimental guy on the block, seeing your mother waving a fully extended condom around on Mother's Day alters the mood of this hallowed occasion just a tad.

As we crossed the street to her house she told me, "I don't know why I did that."

"On Mother's Day you're supposed to sit in your rocker, ponder your Hallmarks, sniff your corsage and sigh," I said.

"I didn't know it was Mother's Day," she said.

A few days later, I drove her back to Cleburne to "check on her house" and visit her sister- and brother-in-law, Olean and Lloyd. She lingered inside her vacant house for two hours, looking over the few things she had left behind during the move. Before we left, she gathered up an armful of tattered newspapers from the 1940s, a coffee mug and some kitchen items, to bring back to her new house in Midlothian. She wanted to visit Raymond's grave "on the way," so we drove the twelve miles in the other direction to Caddo Cemetery between Cleburne and Godley. It's one of the few places that, when she goes there, she isn't ready to leave in five minutes.

That evening, about an hour after I had dropped her off at her new house, she called and said, "Tommy, I'd like to go down to Cleburne tomorrow; you said if I'd move up here you'd take me down there sometime. I heard that somebody's living in my house."

Instead of telling her that we had just gotten back from Cleburne an hour ago and that her house was vacant, empty, untenanted, and otherwise unoccupied, I said, "Do you remember who the neighbors were that lived across the street from us on James Street when I got my thumb cut off?" This happened fifty-five years ago.

"Oh, do you mean Mr. and Mrs. Holley?" she said instantly. "Don't you remember? Mr. Holley took you to the doctor in his Model T. Your thumb was just hanging on by the skin and Daddy held it together till you got to Dr. Cooke's office. You were out in the Stepps' yard playing with Mr. and Mrs. Holley's little granddaughter when you stuck your hand in the mower blades. The Manns lived behind us in an apartment with the Richardsons. The Plummers lived on the other side of the Holleys and Mrs. Powell lived next door to them. She was Mama's friend. Mr. Daly lived in the big house across the street. Everybody called him Grandpa Daly. You broke his pocket watch but he didn't get mad at you. He said it was his fault for letting you play with it. Do you remember that?"

Her memory of the distant past is precise and almost endlessly detailed. She remembers names and places and what people said with pristine clarity—as long as the events took place a long time ago. If I say, "I remember when we had an ice man; he used to chip a fifty-pound block in his truck and carry it inside our house and put it in our icebox," she says:

"That was Leonard Perry. He had that little girl named Connie that you went to school with. Y'all started first grade together. Miss Lula Douse was y'all's teacher. She taught everybody in east Cleburne."

I've learned to turn this ability of hers to my advantage now. Her recent memory is gone. So is, I think, her immediate memory. She can't learn anything new, not even her new address or telephone number. She can dial only a few familiar numbers on the telephone. Her brain is like a short-circuited computer that can call up its old files but no longer saves new material. In this instance, she completely forgot about the Cleburne topic and the hallucination of someone living in her house and didn't return to it—until the next day. Calling up her old files is a simple process and prevents stress.

Thank God for the Good Old Days.

The fact that I didn't know the extent of her disability underscores the oddly distant relationship we've had all my life. If we had spent one day together, just the two of us during the past ten years or so, I would have known. Once, when I took her shopping for a gift, I noticed how easily she wandered away and got lost. When I mentioned this to Raymond, my stepfather and best friend, he deftly switched into his infamous ignore-and-evade mode: "I heard on the scanner that some old woman in the trailer park shot her old husband and drove off to Kansas, pulling the trailer behind her, him still in it. When they found him, he was laid back in his recliner, stiff as a board. Heh, heh, heh." This tactic was effective. Her dotty behavior at Wal-Mart could not compete with the grotesque imagery of Raymond's Johnson County news summaries. I dropped the subject.

But, looking back on it, we can see that there was a benevolent cabal of silence that allowed her to keep her condition hidden, and even the church where she worked was an unwitting conspirator. The truth is, she kept working well beyond the time she should have retired. Despite the good intentions of the church, by allowing her to keep working, it actually helped keep the truth hidden. She must not be too badly off, we assumed, if she can still work. We all knew how unrelentingly Raymond had urged her to quit, but the reason he gave — that her salary caused them to have to pay too much income tax — we now know was only an excuse. He knew she was unable to do the work. When I asked her why she kept working, she always said, "I have a contract I can't get out of." I thought this was one of her little jokes, but she actually believed it. When I finally learned the extent of her disability, I asked her supervisor how she had been able to keep working. She told me that she never left her alone with the children. There had to be someone supervising her as she supervised the children. I assumed that it was out of consideration for her years of devoted service that the church kept her on the payroll.

Though no one can pinpoint the onset of her dementia with very much precision, we in the family learned the extent of it soon after Raymond's death. The most apparent symptom was her fixation on the past and preoccupation with her parents and Raymond as if they were still alive. The present tense is her least favorite grammatical construction. She is generally unaware of her surroundings, and the elements are undeserving of her concern.

She lived in Cleburne when a tornado took out most of South Main Street in 1993. She wasn't in on this news, although she lived less than a mile away. A few months after she moved to Midlothian, another twister ripped past us and smashed Lancaster, a small town twenty miles to the east. There were emergency vehicles on our street with flashing lights, warning everyone to stay inside. I was working that night but called to check on her. The sirens and flashing lights hadn't gotten her attention. "Daddy used to hate storms," she said when I got her on the phone. "He used to get us up out of the bed and make us go down in the cellar. We didn't want to go, but he made us. He had to go down there first and get the snakes out." She went on to enumerate various tempests of her childhood as I tried to wrest from her a description of any damage this particular storm, on this particular evening, might have visited on her present property. It was no use. She was sitting in a storm cellar somewhere in another county in the 1920s.

The news of the world is as a vacuum to her. The last president she remembers is Carter. She is generally oblivious to the usual tabloid travails of important personages in Hollywood, Washington, and London. In fact, if their names don't come up regularly on radio station KCLE in Cleburne, chances are good that she's never heard of them. This station, which plays mainly ancient country music, also has a show called "Trade Fair," a kind of swap meet of the air waves where listeners call in with items to buy, sell, or trade: "I've got an ashtray with Elvis' face in the bottom of it, a thimble collection, with display case, and three dozen fresh-layed eggs, and I'll take five dollars for the whole shebang," says a typical vendor.

This fine show had been number one with Raymond and many other Johnson County devotees for decades. Popular television sitcoms come and go, but "Trade Fair" is forever. If the President of the United States wants my mother's vote, he had better call in to this show and brandish his wares. Since I lean more toward CNN for a somewhat wider, though not necessarily more significant, perspective of world events, I'm hardly "Trade Fair" literate anymore. So when we talk we restrict our conversations to "the Good Old Days."

But even the Good Old Days diversion had its limitations. There was one topic from our past that was profoundly forbidden, a subject I would never bring up, the darkest of family secrets, one never discussed. This unbroachable subject was: What were the circumstances of my birth? Who was my real father, and where was he? Was he really A. B. Dodge, a soldier who had died in the war, as my grandmother said when Brenda asked about him soon after we married? If so, why wasn't I told, so that, if I couldn't know anything else about him, then I could at least know where he was buried? Why was I born?

In short, who am I?

The blackout surrounding this subject was total and absolute. It was as though my mother and grandmother assumed I wasn't interested or, even more amazing, that it had never occurred to me that I was minus a father. I wonder if they lived with the fear that I would bring this discrepancy up someday: "Hey, Mom, you know, I was poking around the house the other day and I just happened to notice something. The old guy in the overalls, outside toiling at his chores, he's the grandfather. Over there, sitting by the window, crocheting, that's the grandmother. There's you, the mother. Then, there's me, the kid. Old Blackie, the family dog—there he is, asleep on the floor. Now, it may just be me, but there seems to be a father missing here. Maybe I'm looking in the wrong places. But if I'm right, then I think you've made a terrible oversight. Somewhere along the way you seem to have misplaced a husband. If it isn't too much trouble, maybe you could busy yourself with the production of this dislocated family member." But the smallest hint that I might raise this question brought the cascading tears.

Of course, they knew how naturally curious I was as a young boy, that I devoured books with the same velocity with which I devoured my grandmother's sugar biscuits. I knew about the lives and doings of great athletes, actors, presidents, explorers, gunfighters, anyone and everyone whose biography rested on the Carnegie Library shelves within reach of my preadolescent, sugar-glazed fingers. Why didn't they know that I was also interested in the identity and life of my own father?

He has been the great hovering void of my life. I always hoped to learn the truth someday, but I didn't think I would ever have the courage to ask my mother about him, or even tell her how this secret has affected me all these years. It was such a painful topic that I could easily justify putting it off, postponing it for another day, another month, another year. Marriage, college, military service, children, grandchildren, a long teaching career and retirement—all came to pass, and this secret remained intact. On occasion, I told myself that one of these days I would find out somehow. Most times, though, I resigned myself to the likelihood that I would never know.

Then, on March 30, 1992, Raymond died. His death changed my back-and-forth attitude toward solving this mystery. It also changed my life drastically and dramatically, though to what extent and to what eventual result I had no way of knowing at the time. It wasn't until I inherited from him the duty of caring for my mother that I learned how far she had actually slipped beneath the waters of this memory-erasing disease, or syndrome, its nomenclature depending on the physician being consulted. Suddenly I was faced with many new and frightening problems, one of which was: even if I ever found the courage to ask her about the mystery surrounding my birth, and if she was willing to talk about it, would she be able to remember? Would her memory of the distant past erode slowly, over a period of months or years, or would it disappear overnight, leaving me with the mystery that no one else in the world could solve?

The doctors I have taken her to assume that she has Alzheimer's, a mental deterioration which can be distinguished from other types of dementia only by an autopsy. Though scientists have traced some forms of it to mutations of genes in chromosomes 14, 19, and 21, knowledge of its cause and cure remains in the future. Its symptoms are recognizable to all whose responsibility it is to care for its victims. My mother's include short-term and immediate memory loss, a lack of facial animation, time confusion, hallucinations, paranoia, delusions, periodic rage, and nocturnal restlessness, plus an assortment of strange or childlike habits. When I think I have seen them all, she springs another one on me.

CHAPTER ONE

We didn't know it when we were kids but Grandpa and Grandma James were separated. Mama never told us. But that explains why Grandma James used to go around and stay with her kids. She'd stay a month with us, then Uncle Jack would come after her and she'd stay with him a month at Blum. Then go from there to stay with all the rest of Mama's brothers and sisters. Us kids always liked to see her coming with that big old trunk. We always wanted to get in it to see what she had in there but she wouldn't let us. Mama got it after she died and then, when she died, it went to me. You'll have it someday. You'd be surprised what all's in there. Grandma James wouldn't let us get in it but she wasn't mean or stingy. She'd give us nickels but she said if she ever caught us getting in her purse she wouldn't ever give us any

*more. She was always thinking that somebody was getting in
her purse. She was a tall woman and would just sit and not
ever say anything till Mama would tap her on the arm and ask
her a question, something about the olden days, and she would
answer and then go back to being quiet again. Mama was
always short. Mama always said she must have got her short-
ness from Grandpa James. Grandpa James was educated and
could keep books. He had the prettiest handwriting, too, and
could play the fiddle. He died when I was little.*

*We used to ask Mama why Grandma and Grandpa James
weren't buried side by side. Mama just said it was because they
wanted Uncle Dock to be buried between them. We found it
out a long time after that they were separated. You didn't talk
about things like that back then. I didn't find it out till after
Mama passed away. I think it was Irene that told me.*

After her initial ten-month attempt to live by herself at
home after Raymond died, a subsequent six-month stay at
a retirement home, and a return to her Cleburne house for
another six months, my mother must have felt like a
delinquent child whose parents moved her from one
school to another when the first sign of trouble developed. But I thought I had to try something else, anything,
to keep her under control but out of a nursing home. I still
believed there was some "perfect solution" to this problem
that would make both of us happy. Helping her became an
obsession with me, and I lost sight of my normal reason.
Even the mystery of my birth became a back-bench issue
during this initial period after we lost Raymond.

During the last few desperate months of her second
attempt to live alone in her Cleburne house, I even considered the possibility of a nursing home for her. The qual-

ity of nursing homes varies, and there are good ones, but I've never seen one I would like living in or one I would want her to live in. Then I noticed that the house across the street from us in Midlothian was available. Why not see about moving her into it? Surprisingly, Brenda was in favor of it, as were the children. Maybe we would just be moving a problem closer to us, I suggested. "At least you won't be gone all the time, back and forth to Cleburne," was Brenda's reasoning.

"Does that house have any foundation problems?" I asked the broker.

"No."

"Any plumbing problems?"

"None."

"Fire ants living in the walls? All the appliances work?" Everything was fine.

"Okay," I said, "I'll take it."

"Don't you want to look at it?"

"I've been looking at it for twenty years. I'm sure it's okay." Ordinarily I can't decide between oatmeal and fried catfish, but with the confidence of a sleepwalker, I uprooted my mother on March 15, 1994, and ensconced her across the street from me.

According to most experts in caregiving, this move would be a mistake. The security of an Alzheimer's victim depends on familiarity and routine, and I had already moved her three times in two years. Although she was desperately lonely and frightened in her Cleburne house (she was calling the police several times every day), she didn't want to move. I didn't tell her that her only other choice was a nursing home. I know she's afraid she's going to end up there. "It's so pitiful," she often told me, "to go out there to the rest home and see all those old people lined up against the walls in their wheelchairs with their heads hanging down." For a while, before the move, even before the plan to move her had formed in my brain, she went through a period of saying, out of nowhere, "Where am I going?" I told her I didn't know why she said such a thing, and she said, "I just feel like I'm going somewhere, maybe that I'm on a waiting list or something." As it turned out, she was right.

The struggle to keep her out of a nursing home hasn't been easy, but it's the choice I've made. When I felt like staying on the canvas and taking the count, I got up and squared off again. I did this, knowing full well of Brenda's uncle, whose refusal to give up his wife to a nursing home until the very last has greatly diminished not only his career as an engineer but his entire life as he knew it before. She began her own descent into the River of Forgetfulness at forty-nine. Now comatose, she lies in a nursing home bed but he remains beside her, caring for her, combing her hair, applying her makeup, as he did before. Though the ordeal has all but broken him, physically and financially, he is still the flag carrier of loyalty and faith. I didn't know whether I had what it took to do this or not.

I didn't even know if it was the right thing, for me. "Look after yourself, too," I was told. "You have a responsibility not only to yourself but to the rest of your family. You can't help her or anyone else if you're in the hospital." I've always had one rule of thumb when it comes to a crisis: I do what I have to do until I can't do it anymore or run out of options. One thing I knew for sure: I was into the short list of options.

At first, after she moved in across the street, I was continually going over there, cooking and doing housework.

Most of the time she was in her bedroom, examining her archives, bank statements from the 1950s and other brittle parchments from the past, relics kept in the old foot locker that once belonged to my great-grandmother James and had become a family icon. It has always held unimaginably valuable treasures: archaic accordion-pleated valentines that opened up to show cherubic cupids aiming their arrows; colored postcards showing luxurious redbrick hotels in Atlanta or Chicago, Louisiana suspension bridges with Model T Fords crossing over them, California redwood trees with highways passing through their gaping, carved-out trunks; greeting cards for all occasions embellished with sentimental or patriotic images long forgotten by our world. Stuffed inside Pangburn candy boxes were hundreds of stiff gray photographs of expressionless men at work beside their farm machinery, at picnics with their women, at fairs and family reunions, and on front porches and beside their automobiles, in studios dressed their best in undersized suits with wing collars and bowler hats, beside dignified, corseted wives with tortured, pinned-up hair, posing mightily in their Sears-and-Roebuck-catalog, post-Edwardian, bulky and brocaded rural finery. Beside them elfin, specter-like children in knickers and homemade shirts buttoned to the chin stood like little stone statues. My grandmother patiently told us who they all were.

There were gray faded daguerreotypes of distant family members, gazing intently across the chasm of generations. Rolled up tightly and tied with ribbons were wide-angle photos of battalions of soldiers in perfect dress-right-dress formation, a tiny X always placed over one head. There were chipped and crumbling war department documents officially and dispassionately chronicling a family tragedy

— namely Uncle Dock's death in the war, from beginning to end. There was a baby's linen dress, tied into a kind of knapsack, holding baby shoes, diaper pins, a lock of hair, and a pair of tiny socks. Just as sacred were Uncle Dock's personal effects: his straight razor, eyeglasses, hymnbook, bow tie, school books, and letters from the war. There were the Liberty nickels that my grandmother said lay on Uncle Dock's eyes. The trunk and its contents were so important that my grandmother left a handwritten note specifying it "must never leave Cleburne." This was her diplomatic way of willing it to my mother, apparently because she was aware of my mother's sentimental need of such a material link to the past.

My mother's obsession with this trunk is profound and absolute. She spends days kneeling before it, sorting through these sentimental totems, these treasured memorials to the only part of her life that isn't threatening. Over the past few years, she has altered its character and composition by adding her own personal treasures. She wraps recent framed family pictures and glass objects — some in bath towels, others in Raymond's underwear — and places them inside the trunk. There seems to be no method in the things she chooses to archive in it. I have found light bulbs in there, ashtrays, kitchen spoons, toothpaste, and even her television clicker — all hidden near the bottom, beneath the archaic family mementos. A clipboard of notes to herself, like "Call and cancel Meals on Wheels," "Call the bank," and "Today is Tuesday," is likely to be found among the treasures. She has opened and closed the trunk lid so many times that she has worn out the hinges.

I have had a recurring dream about that trunk, off and on during my life. It is locked and cannot be opened. I am continually told that there was once a key that opened it and that I am somehow responsible for losing that key. "It's locked in the trunk!" I tell them, but my torturers show no understanding and loom out at me hideously as faces distorted through a fish-eye lens. I know it's in there, but I spend all my time looking for it anyway.

After a while I began to suspect that the many hours she spent on her knees before the trunk, searching through its treasures, might explain her mysterious back pain. She says it's her "sciatical" nerve. Sometimes, she says, the pain is better, but most of the time it's "unbearable." And, always: "Mama had this. It runs in the family."

Three doctors found no real evidence of any back problem. One told me, "It's always something like this. They have a phantom ailment of some kind. Sometimes they just say they're 'weak.' It takes attention away from their real ailment, which they know they have but want to keep anyone else from seeing."

I didn't know what else to do so I got her a dog, a golden retriever named Tipper. She became very fond of him and eventually even learned his name. Tipper lay at her feet and watched as she sorted through her yellowing artifacts. He didn't get despondent about her weirdness or laugh or see anything odd about it at all. If he thought it was strange that she fed him only bread and filled his food bowl with water, he never let on. She kept him in the house and talked to him about her problems. "He knows I have this hurting," she says, "and he knows I'm not putting on."

All of us — Brenda, and children Karen, Lindon, and Lowell — pitched in and decorated her new house with all her familiar things. There were lots of built-in shelves and a built-in china cabinet, which we filled with her

Depression glass collection. We lined the shelves with her family pictures and hung them on the walls in the hall. In her curio cabinet we placed all her small glass figurines.

All of these things soon disappeared. She had taken all the pictures and stacked them in her bedroom closet. All the glass she wrapped in towels and hid under her bed and in the trunk. In her closet she hid all her quilts, her mantle clock, and even the vacuum cleaner.

Her curio cabinet sat in her living room completely empty. Every day she said, "Where are all my pretties?"

"They're under your bed and in your chest where you put them."

"Oh no they're not!"

For the first two or three weeks I played this game. When I would take her into her room and show them to her, she would look at them uninterestedly for a moment, then turn her attention to a youthful picture of Raymond on the shelf. "Didn't Raymond have pretty hair!" she would say.

We couldn't figure it out. Then Brenda, trained as a psychiatric nurse, explained. Her new house is red-and-white brick, the same as the retirement home where she had lived. It has a large family room with a TV, a hallway with bedroom doors on each side, a large dining area with double doors opening into a foyer — all similar enough to cause her confusion.

She stayed in her bedroom most of the time with the door closed, as she had done in her apartment.

She thought she was back in the retirement home!

She was in her new house only a short time before she started telling me about the "old ladies" who lived in the house. "I'm not saying they steal, but I've heard

talk," she whispered in explanation of the hidden possessions.

The "old ladies" talked about her behind her back.
They didn't think she could hear them, but she could.
They said she thought she was "better" than they were
because she's so much "younger" and doesn't have gray
hair. "I heard two old ladies talking the other day," she
said. "One of them said, 'She wears those nice clothes and
gets her hair fixed every week. She thinks she's going to
get a man.' Well, I've got news for them. I don't want a
man. That's the last thing I want. I've never chased a man
and I'm not starting now."

The "old ladies" knew about her "sciatical nerve." They
said: "That lady must be crippled the way she hobbles
around so." Other times, one of them said to the other,
"She must be faking that."

Sometimes, the "old ladies" said she was going to have to
move out because you can't live there if you've been
divorced. This recurring delusion got my attention. I didn't
understand it fully at the time, but I knew it was a clue to
my lifetime of mystery.

I didn't know how to respond to these delusions. At
first I just ignored them. But, sometimes I said, "You
dreamed it." Then, in moments of weakness, I said, "If I
see the old ladies, I'll tell them to leave you alone." The
idea of my reprimanding the old ladies made her happy so
I kept it up. When she brought it up about having to
move, I said, "If they don't leave you alone, we'll just go
up on their rent." She beamed. My opinion was that if she
thought I didn't believe her she might stop talking to me
altogether. She had already accused me of everything
from taking her house away from her to gouging out the
ignition on her car. Brenda said it was better to combat

these delusions, tell her there are no "old ladies" in the house, that it is located in Midlothian, and that we live across the street. So, when I said, "There are no old ladies. You dreamed it," my mother said:

"No, I didn't dream any such thing! They said that when they see you they're going to tell you I've been divorced! But don't you listen to them!"

She talked about the "old ladies" so much that I went out and got one.

It hadn't taken long for us to realize that she needed someone full-time to take care of her, so I advertised in the paper. Karen, our middle child and a natural problem-solver, fielded the virtually endless responses, many from "old ladies" who appeared to need such a service them-selves. She quickly selected Maudie, a quiet and unas-suming woman who cooked, made grocery lists, vacuumed on Thursdays, fed the dog, and watched television five days and nights a week for $175 a week. Maudie served as a companion and my mother liked her, though she often took me aside and whispered, "I don't think Maudie likes me. I heard her tell you that I was lazy."

For the two days and nights each week that Maudie was gone, I had to be Maudie — except for the soap-opera watching. I soon looked toward these two days with dread. I considered hiring someone else to fill in but never got around to it. It would mean that I would have one more "old lady" to worry about. The problem with my mother was getting worse, and the only recognizable end in sight was the end to my patience, energy, and money. Maudie, a fine lady, was left behind in October 1994, when my mother moved back to the retirement home.

The only warning for her episodes of paranoia — "I don't think Maudie likes me" and the constant "gossip" of the "old ladies" — was a sudden look of alarm and urgency in her eyes. When I saw it, I shuddered because I knew she was going to draw me aside and whisper some new tale of conspiracy into my ear. Usually, all I wanted to do was cut the grass or feed the dog in peace without hearing about the "old ladies" and their doings. And I reached the point where I didn't want to hear these shadowy references to the hidden past, which I began to suspect were veiled allusions to the "family secret," if she wasn't going to be specific about them. I was tired of them and made up my mind to press her the next time she brought up the subject. I believed she actually wanted to tell me about my father but was as unable to do it as I was to ask about it.

It came up again while I was trying to attach Raymond's vise to the shelf in her garage. It was hot in there, and the vise weighed over a hundred pounds. I was trying to hold it in place, drill the holes, and bolt it on by myself. She wanted to talk about the old ladies: "They don't like me. They won't quit talking about me."

"What are they saying now?" I managed to utter.

"About my past."

"What about your past?"

"Things they say I've done. I don't have anything to be ashamed of."

"Of course you haven't."

At this point I decided to push further. I stopped what I was doing and said, "Whatever might have happened before I was born, I'd like to know about it. But not from them. You tell them you'll tell me yourself. I'd like to know about it, but only from you. When you're ready."

"There's nothing to tell," she said and went back into the house. The next day she told me for about the tenth time she was going to have to move out because the old ladies said she's been divorced. This time I said: "Have you been divorced?"

"No," she said, looking flustered.

"Then I guess you don't have to move out," I said.

CHAPTER
TWO

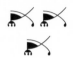

I always thought Raymond
and Lloyd were the two best-looking boys in Cleburne.
Raymond never looked the same after he got his false teeth,
though. He said they never fit right. He used to whittle on
them with his knife. He had to get false teeth because of when
he was in the prison camp they didn't ever get the right things
to eat. He said he had to fight for everything he got. The ones
that couldn't do things for theirselves didn't make it, he said.
He always got an invitation to go to the get-together they had
every year but he just threw it in the trash. He said he didn't
want to have anything to do with the army. And he said if he
ever saw that old captain that surrendered and caused them to
have to be in that old camp he would make him wish he hadn't
done it. He seemed like he was madder at him than he was the

Germans. He said there was one prisoner the guards would kick every chance they got because they thought he was a Jew, but they were never mean to Raymond. Except they took all the things his mother sent him and kept them. He made it, though. Raymond could always take care of hisself.

"Oh, lord, if I wasn't here, she'd starve to death."

That's the nearest Raymond ever came to telling me there was something wrong with her. He said this a few months before he died. There were other hints that I can point to, looking back. "I'll swear, when she puts something up you can't find it to save your life!" He'd say this with utter frustration in his voice as he searched the house for the day's newspaper.

About six months before that, Karen had dropped in on them one Sunday afternoon, and they had been asleep. "Juanita," she said to her grandmother, "did you go to church today?"

She seemed confused and said she hadn't. She asked Karen to call her supervisor and explain that she had "overslept."

She had been there, her supervisor said. My mother started crying when Karen told her she had, in fact, been at work.

Karen was concerned that my mother might be having a stroke and took her immediately to get her blood pressure checked. It was normal. Telling me about it later, Karen said, "Daddy, Raymond sat right there the whole time, knowing she had gone to church, and he didn't say a word."

Karen now thinks he covered everything up because he was afraid we would want to have her put into a nursing home.

Soon after this episode I took her to a psychologist. He gave her a battery of tests and concluded that she was in the intermediate stage of "senile dementia." He said that she would be able to continue for a while doing the things she had been doing for years that required only rote ability, such as dressing, housework, bathing, even working at the church as long as she wasn't expected to learn anything new, or driving as long as she stayed on her familiar route and as long as it was the same car she had always driven. His analysis was somewhat encouraging — and, as we were to learn, unrealistic. At least he didn't say the "A-word," I thought. Plus, there would always be Raymond to see after her.

Unfortunately, though, he hadn't tested her for paranoia. During the drive home, she told me, "They talk about me behind my back down at the church. They think I can't hear them, but I can." I still didn't suspect the severity of the problem. She is forgetful, I thought. They probably do talk about her from time to time. So, I let it go. She's getting older, I reasoned. These things happen. I had my own problems that I thought were so important at the time. And Raymond would always be around to handle everything.

It seems that you'd know it immediately if your mother had Alzheimer's, but she had established our relationship a long time ago and had drawn the boundaries. From my perception, we had always seemed more like siblings separated in age by twenty-one years than mother and son. With no father in my life, I lived with her in my grandparents' house until she got married when I was thirteen. My grandfather's income tax returns for the 1940s and 1950s show both of us as dependents. My grandfather, C. R. Connor, was a father to me. I called him "Daddy" and my grandmother "Ann-A," which was the closest I could come to Annie May as a baby. After I grew up, it was their house we all went to visit and where we gathered for holiday festivities. My children, growing up, spent more time with my mother than I ever did. On weekend visits, they divided their time between her house and my grandparents' house across town. Toward them she was endlessly indulgent. They viewed her as a perfect grandmother.

After my grandparents died in the early 1980s, Brenda took over my grandmother's role of cook on holidays, and everyone gathered at our house. I started going to my mother's house regularly after that, but it was Raymond I spent time with. He did all of the talking, and she stayed in the background. He and I went to my farm. We worked on cars together. He was, by my lights, the world's best mechanic. And, ironically, this greatest of mechanics, this Michael De Bakey of machinery, never made a nickel off of this skill. He was the definitive embodiment of the word "amateur"—he did it strictly for the love of it. He kept not only his cars and lawn mowers running but everybody else's in the family and most of the neighbors' too. I used to sit in one of the old metal lawn chairs in his backyard while he operated on his engines. Talentless in that line, I was fascinated with his genius. His fine steady fingers moved over a clogged carburetor: tiny seals inserted in tiny slots, floats set at the precise level, miniature screws replaced. Shortly, the car was back on the road.

He was the transplant specialist of the machine world. Brushes bad on a generator? No problem. Just remove good ones from a generator with a bent shaft or other severe ailment and transplant them into it. Bypass surgery? He did it thousands of times. Taillights shorted out, and it's too much trouble to track down the problem? He would run a wire directly to the battery and put a small switch on the dashboard to cut them off. Presto. Bypass surgery.

He would figure it out, even if it took weeks. Sometimes, I watched him sitting in his chair, deep in thought about some ornery transmission component or air conditioner compressor or alternator or car window assembly, always something like that. His fingers moved without conscious direction, drawing plans in the air. Then, sooner or later, he would get up and go outside to his workshop and make the broken-down machine work again. He could be slow and methodical, but he never failed.

Carburetors he could set with precision just by listening to the sounds the fuel made as it passed through the chambers. He could eyeball point gaps to a thousandth of an inch. He could even set a car's alignment with a straight cane pole, which he somehow used to measure the toe-in and camber.

Every genius has eccentricities. Raymond cared not a whit for organization or neatness. His garage was a rubble of tools, buckets of parts, small motors, car engines, transmissions, lawn mowers and lawn-mower parts. There were stacks of cigar boxes containing light sockets, breaker switches, gaskets, bearings. Stacks of filters and unopened boxes of spark plugs. Piles of generators, alternators, carburetors, starters, and compressors. Hundreds of belts to pull these parts hung on nails on the walls. Chain saws, hand saws, coping saws, and saw blades. Hammers of every size, clamps, drill presses, even a cast-iron steam engine.

There were literally thousands of such mechanical items, all covered with at least one layer of grease. And fishing equipment, oh lord, it was unbelievable. I found a large grocery sack stuffed with nothing but plastic fishing floats. Another was filled with lures. At one time, he had a full-sized boat inside his garage, and it, too, became a repository of grimy treasures, the bow stacked high with them. His 1963 Volvo broke a motor mount in 1982, requiring pulling the engine in order to replace it, so he parked it inside as well and stacked debris inside it and on top of it for ten years. The rafters swayed with the weight of his collections. Finally, his holdings became so extensive that he could no longer get inside his workshop without squeezing his body between the colossal mounds of rubble. My mother used to say that every time she saw him go in there she was afraid she might never see him again. So, most of the time he could be seen hunkered down, assaying some new treasure outside the door of this impenetrable Fort Knox of junk.

After he died my mother became pathologically obsessed with making sure that not even one screw or washer left that building. She had someone remove the old lock and replace it with a new one, for which she promptly lost the key.

And money. He was funny about money, too. It stuck inside his pockets like Velcro. It wasn't greed. My family could have some of it if we needed it. He never made a dime off of the mowers he piddled with. I've seen him sell mowers to people who actually offered him more for them than he thought they were worth and he would say, "Naw, it's not worth $100. About $75 is a good price for it." He wasn't interested in making a lot of money; he was just interested in holding onto it. He bought what he needed, including clothes, at the flea market. A dollar was about top price he'd pay for a set of spark plugs. He bought items for $50 or less that an ordinary mortal would pay hundreds of dollars for. He usually ended up selling them for only a few dollars more than he paid—and that was after he had repaired them. His pension from a lifetime of working at the Texas Steel Mill in Fort Worth was more than he needed to live on, and he saved the rest. He never bought anything on credit in his life and had no bills except his utilities and taxes. He told me once, "If I wanted to buy something on credit, they probably wouldn't let me do it because I've never had any." Several companies turned me down when I tried to buy insurance on his house after he died because he had never had coverage before. They were suspicious.

When my mother and I were looking through his suits to decide which one to bury him in we found cash stuffed into the lapel pockets like green handkerchiefs. You'd be surprised how much $27,000 stuffed into the lapel pocket can improve the appearance of a polyester, flea-market suit.

My mother used to be very active. She worked at the church or shopped at Wal-Mart or at the mall. She visited relatives and friends in the nursing home. She took Aunt Collie, Raymond's ninety-five-year-old sister, and our Aunt Geneva, my grandfather's youngest sister, to pay their bills. She drove Mrs. Holt, a neighbor, to the bank to check on her money. "Mrs. Holt thinks somebody is getting her money," she used to say, with a laugh.

When she was home, she stayed mostly in the kitchen, cooking her specialty—corn bread and pinto beans and fried sausage. She always had this ready for Raymond and me when we came back from the farm. She was pretty much limited to this menu, but it was always tasty.

Driving was her expertise. And talking to her friends on the telephone.

That didn't include me. We seldom talked. The truth is, I can't remember a single conversation we ever had that lasted over a few seconds. She never asked about what I'd been doing, or how my classes were going. As far as I knew, she didn't even know what I did for a living. If she ever read anything I wrote, she never commented on it. I used to give her copies of my writings but stopped after a while and never mentioned them again when I assumed, rightly or wrongly, that she wasn't interested. Although an only child, I am tortured by sibling rivalry. When a newspaper profile featured me as a local-color radio commentator, the story included a large color photo of me and my cat with my great-grandfather's antique icebox in the background.

Eternal hope for recognition from her roiled in my breast. I showed her the article.

"Oh, gracious!" she cried, gazing adoringly at the photo. "Would you look at that! Isn't that something!"

By this time I'm swelling up like a leaky pipe. I can't believe it! These breathless accolades—after all these years!

"There's Grandpa Conner's icebox!" she says. "Right there in the paper! I can't wait to show this to Aunt Geneva!"

"Well," I say, "do you see anything else in the picture that you recognize? Anything?"

"Oh, yeah," she says. "Well, sure I do. There's the cat."

"Yeah," I say, "the cat. Anything else? What about the person in the picture? Does he look familiar?"

"Well, he looks a little like you. Except he's not quite as fleshy. What's he doing in your kitchen?"

It wasn't all her fault. Communication requires two people. Raymond was easier to talk to, and I could be sure that he wasn't going to start crying if the conversation turned toward a topic more serious than the price of paper towels at Wal-Mart. I never once considered her feelings when I promptly asked for him when she answered the phone. That she trained me as a child to avoid serious conversation with her is a poor excuse for my failing at least to ask her how things were going before saying, "Is Raymond there?"

CHAPTER THREE

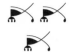

Mama used to have the asthma so bad. You remember that, don't you? You called her "Ann-A" because you couldn't say Annie May. After a while Daddy started calling her that, too. She was still suffering with it after we moved over on English Street. It used to scare us when we were kids. We used to look at her and cry, the way she was straining to breathe. We thought she was going to die. But I think she began to get better after old Dr. Cooke gave her that stuff in the can that she burned. She used to get under the tablecloth and breathe the smoke. It came in a green can. It was like dry leaves. Sometimes she'd let us get under there with her. You used to like to get under there with her, too, when you got big enough. Before she got that, Daddy would get up with her in the night and wash her face with cold water till she got to where she could breathe. Dr. Cooke was a good doctor. He never charged anything. He would take the money if you offered it, but he never sent a bill.

Mama couldn't get around cotton without it happening. That's why we couldn't stay at Lubbock. She was sick all the time. Aunt May and Uncle Den stayed and we came back. I was glad. At first we were living in an old barn that didn't even have a floor. I wanted to get back to Cleburne.

That was when we moved to that sandy-land farm east of Cleburne. I used to spend the night with friends that lived down the road from us. That would be Mary Bess and Vera. They were sisters. There was another one named Fritz — she was Bernice's friend — and one they called Peggy. She was a lot younger. She was the prettiest little girl I ever saw. I always thought all of those girls were the prettiest girls I ever saw and wore the prettiest clothes. They had a nice, big old house. Their daddy had been a warden at a prison and they always had a lot of money. They had two brothers, Tommy and Johnny. I used to go out on dates with Tommy. He was so good looking. And Bernice went with Johnny. Mostly, we just went to church. After we moved to town we kept on going out there. You used to listen to the ball game with their daddy, but he made you mad when he said he wouldn't listen to Gordon McLendon because he had beer commercials.

Daddy quit farming before the war and moved to Cleburne. I guess it was because Coon and Wayne had left home about that time and he couldn't get the crops in by hisself. Coon was always his favorite, I think, but he used to whip the daylights out of him. Mainly for cussing. When we moved to town we lived at 1202 East James. Daddy went to work for the WPA and made a dollar a day. He didn't like not farming anymore but he was proud we didn't have to go on relief like a lot of other people. He chopped cotton and helped build ballparks and swimming pools. He always said he worked on the WPA with Ernest Tubb. He said Ernest just threw his hoe down one day and walked off. He said he wasn't ever going to hoe another row of cotton as long as he lived. Daddy said he should have stuck with it. He could hoe a lot better than he could sing. It was the first time we had ever lived in town. I liked being able to work and make money without having to pick cotton. I kept house for an old couple that lived over on Poindexter. I made two and a half a week. I'd take that two and a half and buy me a new pair of shoes. But it didn't take long to wear out a pair of shoes walking all the way over there and back every day. There were lots of stores close enough to walk to when I wanted to buy things. When I worked at Duke & Ayres and Woolworth I thought I was rich. We had running water and even had an ice man. His name was Leonard Perry. We weren't used to having neighbors so close either. We liked them all—the Stepps, the Dalys, the Holleys, the Hubbards, the Powells, and the Plummers. The Manns lived behind us.

The Meltons lived in the house next door. The Manns lived behind us and the Hubbards lived on the corner. Mrs. Rogers lived across the street. She was a grouchy old lady. You used to go through the fence to the Meltons' house and Mr. Melton would give you relief apples. You weren't but about two years old. You used to go all over that neighborhood. We didn't worry about you. We knew you'd come back home when you got hungry. Mama used to give you biscuits with butter and sugar on them. You were a mess. You dropped Mama's wedding ring through a hole in the floor and we never could find it. You weren't old enough to tell us what you did with it. When you learned to talk you told us. By that time we had already moved over on English Street and somebody else was living there. Mama didn't blame you though. She just said she had no

*business letting you play with it. Little things like that didn't
matter to her because she had been through so much.*

For intimacy growing up I read books.

At ten years old, I started my book collection. I saved
up $10 and bought my own bookcase, which I still have.
It was always important to me to have books. My grandfather couldn't read or write. My grandmother read only the
Bible and the *Cleburne Times Review.* My mother read
Photoplay, Modern Screen, and *Hollywood Confidential.* If
she thought my early literary interests were good or bad,
she never said. Is there such a thing as a reading gene and,
if so, where did mine come from? My mother's recent
veiled references to the hidden secret of my father plagued
me. For the first time in life, I began to suspect that A. B.
Dodge might not be my real father at all. I didn't look at
all like him, and his driver's license showed him to be a lot
smaller. Was he only the "beard," a convenient cover-up,
or stand-in, for someone else, a married man, maybe, with
a book collection?

I came to be suspicious of anyone she had known
named Tommy. After Raymond died she began bringing
up an old boyfriend with what I considered conspicuous
regularity. His name is Tommy, and he's still alive. They
were neighbors when they were teenagers, and she and
Aunt Bernice, her younger sister, used to double-date
with him and his brother. He went on to become a major
league baseball player. I looked him up and gave him a
call. He works in a bookstore in San Antonio! This was
the one! I thought. I had a bookstore once. As a baseball
fan, I have no peer. Where was this book-loving baseball
player nine months prior to February 12, 1939?

I had known about him all my life and had always wanted to write a feature on him. He was one of the three major league players associated with Cleburne, Spike Owen and Tris Speaker being the other two. This was a perfect time to do it. He turned out to be a genial man with a relaxed manner and expressive vocabulary. He asked about my mother and said they had gone out on dates when they were teenagers.

"When did you leave Cleburne?" I asked.

He left in 1937. This would be too early to make him a prime suspect, although he could have returned on visits. Romantic reunions, you know. He was number one on my list of possibilities.

I was almost grown before I consciously realized that my mother and I had an odd relationship. She never came to see me in school plays and on the baseball team, never gave me a birthday party, never took me to one, or made me a cake. If there were any birthday cakes, my grandmother made them, just as she made my costumes for school plays. My mother worked, though, and was generous with the little money she made. The money she gave me financed my enormous craving for comic books and tickets to the Texas and the Palace, movie theaters where western stars Gene Autry and Roy Rogers and all the lesser-lights of the Saturday matinee lit up my heavenly fantasy world with six-guns, silver saddles, and sagebrush serenades. When I complained of having to hitch a ride to the movies with my friends on their bikes, she bought me a new Western Flyer from Western Auto. She bought it on credit and when, filling out the loan form, the salesman said, "Your husband's name?" she said,

"I don't have one."

Don't have one? Why not? I remember thinking, how

can this be? Does this mean I was born without a father? I'm actually glad I hadn't been to Sunday school enough to have known about immaculate conception. In my college Greek classes no other student searched out the derivation of the word "parthenogenesis" with more enthusiasm.

My grandmother was well trained as an accomplice in this conspiracy of silence, though she lacked the talent for embellishment. She never discussed the fact that her own parents had lived apart because, I'm sure, her mother never discussed it with her. Like mother, like daughter. My grandmother had the strength to bear any tragedy, but scandal was indefensible. These women didn't try to put the best face on scandal; they didn't put any face on it at all. Their pride was beyond all understanding when judged by today's standards. Though they weren't ashamed to be poor, they placed great store by the fact that they never had divorces, never had trouble with the law, and never went on relief—called welfare today. But nothing was more dreaded than scandal.

When Brenda first came into the family, my grandmother told her, "Tommy's daddy was named A. B. Dodge, and he's been dead a long time." That was it.

Ann-A's handicrafts were everywhere in her house. Latticed patterns of intricate design covered the backs of every chair and every arm. Up and down, this way and that, around and up, back and around again, her fingers, like spinnerets, guided the thread precisely through tiny interlacing loops. She did it without thought. It was like magic. Only rarely did an error occur. Then, she would back up a few stitches, inspect the work momentarily, make the correction, then go at it again, ninety miles an hour, as if to make up the lost time. Soon, the balls of colored thread in her lap were transformed into these masterworks of furniture art, seemingly as varied and intricate as snowflakes.

Each bed was covered by a bedspread from her needle and sagged with the weight of her handcrafted quilts, and all the closets bulged with them. She made the curtains, the rugs, and the tablecloths. In her quilts we all recognized patches of our clothing, having served its purpose on our backs, now artfully recycled for extended utility. Nowadays, she would be called a "folk artist."

She made all her own clothes, many of my mother's and mine, even my underwear, until I was in junior high school. This school was located in the west or "rich" part of Cleburne. I soon learned that the kids who went to this school didn't wear homemade clothes. Their parents bought them at stores. I wanted this, too. With her small Woolworth salary—$22 a week—my mother hardly managed to afford the material for her own clothes, lunches at the Ace Cafe, and reading material and movie tickets for me. My new clothing expense was impossible for her and hard for my grandfather, too, on his laborer's paycheck from the Santa Fe shops. A pair of Levis in those days cost $3.85. For that amount of money, my grandmother could probably have made five pairs of pants. But they managed to buy them for me because they raised most of our food in the large garden spot behind our house and didn't waste money on a car, a television, indoor plumbing, or even soap. My grandmother made her own lye soap from the fat she saved from the kitchen. It didn't lather very well but got clothes clean, and me, too, and my mother said it was good for your hair. By the time I was in high school we had store-bought soap and these other luxuries, too.

Any upbringing I might have had I owe to my grandparents. They were as unconditional in their love as they
were undemonstrative in the display of it. Though they
weren't affectionate to one another, to me, or to anyone
else, they never argued or quarrelled and never punished
me. They went to church together, to gospel "singings,"
shopped, and worked together in the garden. The affection they felt for each other was apparent in subtle ways
to those who knew them, especially in the way they
worked together in the garden. It was like a choreo-
graphed dance—he picking corn and pulling up onions,
slapping them against his pants leg to knock off the dirt,
she in her apron and bonnet, moving alongside a few rows
away, snapping beans into a basket that she dragged along
behind her.

I used to love going out to the garden and following
along behind my grandfather as he pushed his plow, feeling the cool and moist black dirt under my bare feet.
Then, later, going out to help bring in okra, beans and
peas, potatoes, onions, mustard and turnip greens,
spinach, beets, and ears of corn. Until my cousin
Durwood, Uncle Coon's son from Los Angeles, came to
visit one time, I thought every kid did this. I took him out
to the garden to help me pull some ears of corn and shuck
them for supper. Looking at the silk, he said, "How do you
get this hair off of them?" Soon after Brenda and I were
married, I asked her to go out to the garden and bring in
potatoes for supper. She came back and said, "There's not
any left. There's not a single potato on those vines!"

My mother's ecstasy had nothing to do with garden soil
between her toes, however. Neither did her joy include
helping my grandmother with her cooking, or learning to
crochet, quilt, or raise chickens. She liked to work in

retail stores, buy clothes, socialize with her friends, and go to Clark Gable movies.

She ate with us on Sundays but did no more than I did to help my grandmother prepare the meal. Her job was to wash dishes and clean up. She still enjoys doing this. My job was to watch my grandmother. First, she selected a nice fryer to have a sizzling rendezvous with a cast-iron skillet. Sometimes, on special occasions like Thanksgiving, she picked a fat hen out of the flock. "All right, old sister," she would say as she backed her prey, now clucking the cluck of the condemned, up against the shed, "I told you if you didn't lay you'd go in the pot." Soon, she had the hen by the head and, after a few revolutions, she held only the head in her hand. Its dull, unblinking eye seemed always to be fixed on me. Ann-A wrung a hen's neck with no more emotion than if she were winding a watch. The old sister flopped around on the ground for a while, till all its blood was gone, pumped out through the exposed spinal cord. Sometimes, I would come home from school and know we were having chicken for supper because my grandmother's ankles would be caked with dried blood. Then, into the boiling water of her cast-iron pot it went, to soften the quills for easy plucking. The feathers were saved for later use in pillows and mattresses. After that, the old sister was cleaned and cut up, baked and stuffed with the most divinely inspired corn bread-and-biscuit dressing ever concocted by mortal hands. Add to that a big bowl of new potatoes, roasting ears, mustard greens, green beans, plenty of cat-head biscuits, chocolate pie and banana pudding, and you had a meal to rival any of those described in a Thomas Wolfe novel, a feast so delectable it barely left us with the power of respiration. Locomotion, for a considerable period of time thereafter, was out of the question. Anyone who has ever been blessed with the access to such sublime cookery understands without explanation that old cliche, "you can't go home again."

August meant grape jelly. Picking mustang grapes might not appeal to modern boys, but for me it was a grand adventure, to be compared with a trip to Six Flags for a young boy today. Because she was allergic to the vines, my grandmother prepared for the occasion by dressing in one of my grandfather's long-sleeved shirts, thick stockings, gloves, and bonnet. Then we fetched our baskets and set out for the land where the wild vine grows.

To get to where the grapes were, we had to crawl through a fence and follow Buffalo Creek for a long way until it widened into a swimming hole deep in the woods. The kids called this place "Grapey," because high trees formed a canopy over it full of mustang grape vines. The older boys swung on them and dropped into the water.

Almost always full of naked boys on these boiling August afternoons, the scene looked like an Eakins painting. I wasn't allowed to go into the water because I hadn't learned to swim. But, one day, as we were picking grapes nearby, I could hear the boys splashing and making joyful cries, and I begged my grandmother till she said I could go over and watch. I wouldn't go in, I promised.

I left her to fill the baskets and ran through the vines till I came to where my friends were. They were all very old, at least thirteen. I sat on the bank for a while, watching their fun. I remembered my promise, but it was hot, and the water was so cool. Maybe I could have resisted if they hadn't started double-dog-daring me. I didn't like the idea of breaking my promise but, when I made it, I had no idea that double-dog-dares were going to get involved.

Pretty soon, my clothes lay in a pile on the bank and I was swinging through the air on a vine high over the water. I was a Flying Wallenda! I was Tarzan! My friends were treading water below, yelling for me to turn loose.

An inexperienced Tarzan, I held on too long and hit the edge of the bank when I dropped. When I crawled up on the bank, my foot was bleeding, the soft flesh laid open to the bone by a sharp rock.

Some of the boys helped me get my clothes on and the others went to get my grandmother. She tore a piece off of her shirt and wrapped my foot to slow down the bleeding. It was a long way back home, but the boys took turns carrying me on their backs and carrying the full baskets of grapes. My foot hurt, but not as much as my conscience for going back on my promise.

When we got home my grandmother went to the shed and got a fruit jar full of kerosene, which she called coal oil, and used it to clean out the deep cut. My friends watched, wide-eyed, and each later told his own version of the dramatic event.

The next morning I looked out of my bedroom window and saw smoke rising from underneath the iron kettle. This meant she was cooking the grapes. When they were ready she dipped out the mixture and separated the juice from the pulp by squeezing it all through cheesecloth. Then she cooked it some more and added about five pounds of sugar and some things that made it thicken. Before long we had several hot jars of purple nectar. By the time it cooled it would be jelly. My foot, and my conscience, still throbbed, but I knew that my grandmother's hot biscuits packed with her homemade mustang grape jelly could take your mind off of just about anything.

I'm sorry to say this wasn't the last time I ever broke a

promise and gave in to peer pressure. She never condemned me for this, though. Her favorite expression in
the face of such failure was, "We all fall short of the glory
of the lord." These soft words, and a full belly of my
grandmother's biscuits and mustang grape jelly, could, I
believed, reform the heart of the most hardened criminal.

My mother's apparent indifference to all things domes-
tic and virtually everything other than her job at the five-
and-dime, her friends, and romantic movies, extended to
my school work also. I still have all my report cards from
elementary school. During those first six years I never
made any grade less than perfect in all subjects, even con-
duct. She always signed them and handed them back to
me without comment of any kind. I thought everybody
made perfect grades. She signed them "Juanita Dodge," a
name I would later learn she had no legal claim on but
one she appropriated to protect us all from social stigma.

I was in the second or third grade before I realized there
was something unusual about my family. All my friends
had one mother, one father and, usually, brothers and sisters. One day on the playground after school, a friend said,
"My mother said you're a bastard and your mother is a
whore."

I knew vaguely what those words meant, though I'm
not sure my friend did. My face burned as though it was
on fire and I started crying. I ran all the way from the
Santa Fe Elementary playground to his house, about half
a mile away, with him running along beside me saying,
"I'm sorry! I'm sorry!" I was almost out of control when I
ran into his house and screamed at his mother:

"Why did you say that? Why did you say that?"

She was calm and her explanation was soothing, but I
didn't get over it for a long time. She said, "All anybody

ever knew was that your mother went to Houston and came back with you." This woman was a good person and otherwise treated me nicely. "We all fall short of the glory of the lord." My childhood friend is still a close friend, but we don't talk about this incident. I hope he has forgotten it.

Until 1969, when I located the man said to be my father, my friend's mother's explanation, cruel as it was, was all anyone ever gave me.

CHAPTER
FOUR

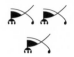

Cleburne didn't used to be like it is now. It was like a carnival downtown on Saturday night. All the stores stayed open till nine and everybody parked their cars and walked up and down the sidewalks, looking at the window displays. Kids drove their cars around and around the square, the ones that had them did. There were six or seven drugstores and lots of grocery stores, three picture shows, lots of dress shops and shoe stores, and either a barber shop or a cafe on every corner. Morris Neal had that little hole-in-the-wall hamburger joint—right there next to where Packwood's Barber Shop used to be—it had a little window there facing the alley where you could just drive through and get six hamburgers for a dollar and six doughnuts for a quarter and never have to get out of your car. If you had *a car. We had to walk up to the window and get ours because we didn't have a car.*

And Woolworth! It was like Grand Central Station in there. After I started working downtown you used to come to town on Saturday night with Mama and Daddy. Daddy would buy his groceries at Ted Burd's, and Pee Wee Randolph would give y'all a ride home. It was fun back then.

Daddy got a job moving houses for old T. D. Nutt and was able to get off the WPA. Daddy called him "Old Nutt." He was a big old fat guy with a big nose. He used to give you buffalo nickels. After that Daddy went to work for the Quartermaster Depot in Fort Worth, during the war. Don't you remember? He had to get up at three in the morning to go to work. He used to ride with Shorty Clack. Shorty killed hisself because he had those bad headaches. After the war Daddy got laid off at the Quartermaster. That's when he got on at the railroad. Things started getting better after that.

Cleburne, the county seat of Johnson County, is located thirty miles south of Fort Worth. It gets its name from Confederate General Patrick Cleburne. Civil War historian Shelby Foote places him next to Lee, Grant, and Sherman as the most interesting military figures of that war. He was the first officer to recommend allowing slaves to earn their freedom by fighting in the war.

Throughout most of my childhood, the city limits signs placed the town's population at 10,558. Though the Santa Fe Railroad was the backbone of Cleburne's economy, the town was also known for its farms and dairies, cattle, football teams, churches, and bootleggers. As far as Cleburne is concerned, the Volstead Act is operative to this day. My grandfather used to say that more people died in car wrecks going to Fort Worth for liquor than ever died from drinking it.

English Street, a short, unpaved street running parallel to Henderson Street on Cleburne's east side, hasn't changed much in appearance since those days of my grow-ing up—dusty hackberry and chinaberry trees and small frame houses owned by working-class families and vacant lots that neighbors plow up in the spring to plant gardens. Like most other men in our neighborhood, my grandfa-ther worked for the Santa Fe, which he called the "Sainty Fee," a pronunciation typical of his unorthodox lingo (but historically sound, as I would later discover). In 1989, the Santa Fe abandoned the town after a hundred years of operation there. Its repair shop had been the largest of its kind between Galveston and Kansas City, for many years maintaining and repairing more than 500 engines and 6,000 boxcars each year.

Since the turn of the century there was but one destiny for most of the boys growing up on Cleburne's east side: you followed in your father's oily footsteps at the railroad. Though you usually got off from work as grime-faced as a coal miner, you were paid as much as the boys on the other side of town with their college degrees or jobs in their fathers' stores or factory offices or banks. Engineers· earned as much as some doctors or lawyers, bought new cars every other year, never had to get dirty,. and were respected in the community. Working at the Santa Fe I made $2.26 an hour as a teenager when the minimum wage was less than a dollar. In my last year as a fireman, for the Texas & Pacific, in 1964, I made $6,000, and engi-neers made twice that. My friends who stayed on after I left now earn $65,000 or more as engineers. Between the years 1904 and 1984, when the Santa Fe began its leave-taking, it was the lifeblood of the town's economy. In 1950, the shops employed 1500, had a payroll of $6 million and paid $50,000 in taxes to the city on its 232 acres of land. Based on an average family of four, this meant that over half the town's population depended directly on the railroad for its livelihood. In that year the Santa Fe paid my grandfather $62.50 a week. In 1984, its last big year, the shops employed 750 workers and had a payroll of $21 million. Workers repaired and maintained 638 locomotives, and its yard crews operated the forty trains a day that passed over its sixty-seven miles of shop tracks. It had its own fire department, where my grandfather worked, its own water system of six wells producing 850,000 gallons of aquifer water a day, and its own hospital at Temple, the best there was, my grandfather said.

At the intersection of East Henderson and Border stood Cleburne's train station and depot, built in 1894, said to be Texas' finest on the Gulf, Colorado & Santa Fe line. Actually there were three depots there at one time. Behind the Santa Fe depot, across Border Street to the west, was the depot for the Trinity & Brazos Valley line (also known as the "Boll Weevil" because during the Depression it carried cotton farmers to and from Austin as they sought government help to eradicate the boll weevil). And, on the east side, across the tracks, was the Missouri, Kansas & Texas (the "Katy") depot. When this line folded the depot became a feed store, which burned a few years ago. The Trinity & Brazos Valley depot became an antique store with that line's demise and it, too, later burned.

The Santa Fe passenger station covered the whole block from Henderson back to Chambers Street toward the south where it housed the yard office and a Harvey House restaurant of the chain begun in 1876 by Fred Harvey in a Santa Fe depot in Topeka, Kansas. The waitresses, known as "Harvey Girls," wore black uniforms and white aprons. They lived upstairs and were required to remain unmarried for one year and not socialize with the trainmen. Many of them fell in love and got married within a few months, however. The Harvey House closed in 1931 and the station burned ten years later. When it was rebuilt the top floor was left off and the building was given a more modern look. On the north side of Henderson was another building used for baggage storage and handling. Hungry passengers and trainmen either walked across to the Harvey House or boarded a horse-drawn cab and rode the few blocks downtown. I can remember passengers waiting for connections in a little park once located there. My mother remembers the YMCA. building located just to the north of the park. It was a stately three-story red-brick building with white trim and two large verandas where guests could sit out-side and watch the trains' arrivals and departures. On the lawn were two tennis courts. Besides its twenty bedrooms, it had a library, gymnasium, bath houses, bowling alley, basketball court, and a spacious, luxurious lobby. At one time it had a membership of over a thousand, the largest in the state.

Just a block further north were the Santa Fe shops. The most notable landmark was its 213-foot smokestack, near the east gate. It was built in 1929 and is still the tallest structure in the city. No matter where you are in town you can see the smokestack. It is fourteen feet in diameter and sunk seventeen feet into the ground. I never saw smoke coming out of it. I hope somebody doesn't think of a good reason to dynamite it down some day, but I suspect they will.

The smokestack was always associated in my mind with the whistle. When we were growing up, my cousins visiting from the Gulf coast always said, "the boats are coming in" when the whistle blew three times a day. The whistle now belongs to the Age of Steam Railroad Museum in Dallas.

Cleburne still has a large population of retired railroaders, many of them fathers of my classmates. They live well on good pensions and have excellent medical coverage. They still buy their share of new cars and otherwise contribute to the town's economy, or what is left of it. To my mind they represent a kind of ideal life that is disappearing in a world of encroaching alienation. Their sense of fraternal bond, comradeship, and community loyalty is almost unknown elsewhere in corporate America. Most of them still live and breathe railroading. But those I worked with, their sons, won't be retiring in Cleburne. They've had to relocate, or take buy-outs. In a few years, the last of the old guard of Cleburne's railroading days, like the depots, the repair shops, the YMCA, the Harvey House, and the Santa Fe Park, will all be gone.

As a boy I lay in my bed late at night and listened to the sound of the boxcars bumping together in the train yard and the wailing of the whistle as the freight trains passed the East Henderson Street crossing. They were ghostly but comforting sounds, ones that east side Cleburne boys won't be hearing ever again with that same heart-quickening happiness I felt in knowing that the trains were running in Cleburne and all was right with the world. I still dream about those trains.

With the Santa Fe gone, many of the houses along East

Henderson Street where our friends lived have been transformed into restaurants, used car lots, and antique shops. Now, when we drive down this street, my mother says, with hardly a variation, "There's where Dr. Bell used to be. I used to walk up here to his office when I had a toothache. There's old Willie Randolph's store. Before he was there, Alice Williams had a store in an old clapboard house. There's Hub Booth's house. I used to work at Woolworth's with Dorothy Booth. Do you remember when she threw that pan of scalding water through the window screen into old Skyblue's face because he was peeping at her? There's Shorty and Burnice's store. You and old Blackie used to go up there every day and get lunch meat and Cokes. There's the Rothmells' house. Those old ladies used to keep that place spic and span. Now look at how it's all junked up. It was the prettiest house on the street. They were Germans. There's where Jesse and Carrie lived and the Petersons. Do you remember Mr. and Mrs. Finley? We just passed where their house used to be. Mr. Finley used to break up our garden with his old horse. The old horse's name was Buck. LaDell Reeves married their daughter. He's our cousin. Otis Peterson's house sure has gone down. The Procks' house don't even look like itself, painted yellow like that. Our old house is sure junked up. It never looked like that when we lived there."

She gets quiet around the time when we come to where the railroad tracks crossed East Henderson (there's an overpass there now) and doesn't start up again till we get to where the Central Texas Bus Line used to be. Then she recollects all those days when we used to ride the bus to Joshua every Sunday to spend the day with Grandpa Conner and how Lindon and Lowell and Karen used to ride it from Midlothian every weekend when they were little. We turn the corner and go two blocks and she says, "There's the church. Mary Beth is in there taking care of the kids. She got my job. They gave her a little raise."

In the summers back in the days she remembers so vividly, the town always seemed to yawn and put its feet up. She and the other women of the neighborhood sat on the wide front porches in their summer dresses and swatted flies and chatted about the boys who came back from the war and the ones who didn't, of getting up at three in the morning to stand in line at Burr's Department Store to get a pair of nylon hose, about rationing coupons and what it would be like to have all the chocolate you wanted. Sometimes the others knitted and crocheted to the dramatic vicissitudes of "Stella Dallas" and "Just Plain Bill" as the plaintive sounds of these early-day radio soap operas wafted through the screen door.

With the neighborhood boys I ran the summer-evening gauntlet of lawn sprinklers as we chased around the yards and pulled one another down to the cool wet grass. We lay on our backs and looked up at the night sky. Without city lights and pollution to obliterate it, the Milky Way was spread out above us like a canopy of whipped cream. It looked close enough for you to reach up and scoop off a handful. My grandmother said it was leftover stars that God hadn't gotten around to separating yet. In college I learned that the Greek poet Homer's version ran counter to her explanation. He said that a pregnant goddess squeezed her swollen breasts and spewed milk across the sky. My grandmother would never have repeated such a theory.

I had a Captain Midnight Secret De-Coder ring and a Lone Ranger pedometer. I had no idea what a pedometer was. But I sent the Cheerios boxtops and the $2 because the Lone Ranger said to do it, and the Lone Ranger never steered you wrong and was to be obeyed.

My life was further embellished by marbles, pocketknives, homemade slingshots, dog and horse books by Thomas C. Hinkle, Texas tales by J. Frank Dobie, numerous readings of Huckleberry Finn and Tom Sawyer, Robin Hood, Robinson Crusoe, the Hardy Boys mysteries, frequent visits to the Carnegie Library for extended perusals of archived newspaper accounts of historical events and box scores of classic baseball games, and a continuum of comic books with their array of spectacular heroes. Summer afternoons meant lying on my bed with the radio tuned to KLIF and the Old Scotsman's Liberty Broadcasting Company and his dramatic renditions of the baseball game of the day. He had a magnificent voice with grand and exaggerated inflections and a naturally cadenced delivery. Metaphors and allusions from the classics, from baseball's antiquity, and from his boyhood farm life, enlivened and enriched his description of the action on the field. He was an orator of baseball, the William Jennings Bryan of the broadcast booth. His opening remarks went something like this:

"Play ball with the Liberty Broadcasting System! Hello everybody everywhere, this is the Old Scotsman, Gordon McLendon, bringing you the game today from Yankee Stadium, the House that Ruth Built, between the New York Yankees, the Ruppert Rifles, and the second-place Boston Red Sox, led in this pennant race by the amazing Ted Williams, the Kid, the Thumper, the Splendid Sprinter, last player in the major leagues to hit .400, a sterling batsman, who will look as dangerous up there at the plate to Yankee pitcher Whitey Ford today as the legendary Achilles looked to Hector on the windy plains of Troy."

And on like that. The Old Scotsman was one of my real-life heroes. For lonely imaginative boys, yearning for some desperate glory, he manufactured great fantastic images of heroes like Ted Williams, Joe DiMaggio, Bob Feller, Van Lingle Mungo, and a pantheon of other players built up in my mind to a size far beyond mortal proportions. From the Old Scotsman I also learned baseball history. On Mondays, when the teams were traveling, he picked a classic game from baseball's past and, simply by looking at the scoresheets found in back issues of the *Sporting News*, re-created the game with the art of a stage magician.

In fact, they were all re-created. The Old Scotsman was in his radio studio in downtown Dallas, getting the action of the game off the wire. For added verisimilitude, he sent sound crews to all the ballparks, so that when Jackie Robinson stole home, the roar of the crowd had a Flatbush accent. To simulate the sound of the bat striking the ball, he thumped a bat suspended on a string with a pencil. When there was a breakdown in the tickertape, he filled in with stories of baseball's past, a talent for which he had no equal. There are no parallels to him among today's announcers. I guess I was addicted to his broadcasts. My mother used to say, "No need to ask Tommy to do anything. He's got to listen to Gordon."

Many years later I sent him a copy of a sports book I had done, and he called me up. He was a multimillionaire by then, a kind of benevolent power broker, having invested in radio stations, drive-in theaters, real estate and strategic metals. We became friends, and I wrote several speeches and voice-over narrations for him until he was hit by cancer and died in 1986. In 1984, I wrote a piece called "The Old Scotsman and the Ghost of Baseball Past," which was included in a sports anthology. I was to read it at a sports convention at San Diego State University, but it looked as though this would be impossible, as the college where I was teaching rejected my travel proposal to read an article about "sports." I mentioned this to the Old Scotsman. A couple of days later, travel funds came flying in from all directions around campus, from sources I hadn't even known about. The next time I saw the Old Scotsman, he peered at me over his glasses and said, "Things going better for you out at the college?"

CHAPTER FIVE

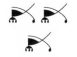

My cousin John Brown moved us over to English Street in his truck. We didn't have a bathroom in that house either, just an old privy outside. Whoever lived there before us left two greyhounds and you fed them relief hominy that you found in one of the old sheds. You loved living over there because you could go next door to the Walkers' house and listen to all their tall tales. You came home one time and said that there was such a thing as radios with pictures on them where you could see things that were happening a long way off. You said you heard Shorty Walker talking about this with some of his buddies.

You used to come home with some of the biggest stories that you heard in the neighborhood. When you weren't at the Walkers' house you were at the Flippens'. I didn't like for you to go down there either, because they let that little old Flippens boy smoke cigarettes and he couldn't have been over six years old. There was always something happening down there. Like the time the Flippens girl ran off with some boy and her mother found her and drug her back home — there you were, right in the middle of all the ruckus. I think it was Dorothy's little sister — Dorothy was the red-headed one that was married to Bootle. Wayne used to laugh at your stories about Bootle. That time when the creek got up and like to have washed us all away, there you were down there with the Flippens again. They were going to run away from it. They had Bootle's old car all loaded up with every-thing in the house and then there wasn't any room for him because he weighed about three hundred pounds. So Dorothy said, "Get in the turtle, Bootle darlin'!" Wayne thought that was about the funniest thing he ever heard. But old Bootle was good to you. He used to sit out on the front porch and play his guitar and sing, and you and Billy Wayne and Darrell thought Bootle hung the moon. Then all those big war stories he used to tell y'all. You used to come home and tell all that. About shooting the Japs' legs off and they kept right on coming on their stumps. I never heard such windy stories. Those were hard old times but we didn't know it. We had fun.

As the Old Scotsman's sonorous tones and dramatic inflections filled my little sugar-biscuit brain with excite-ment and wonder, the summer breezes fluttered the leaves on the hackberry trees outside my bedroom window, and the white leghorn hens and the dominickers bock-bock-bedocked in the backyard. At night I went to sleep listen-ing to the likes of Bob Hope, Fred Allen, Red Skelton, *The*

Easy Aces, Dr. I.Q., Your Hit Parade, with Frank Sinatra and Eileen Wilson, and, on Saturday nights, *The Grand Ole Opry.*

In those days there were small, friendly, neighborhood grocery stores, filled with the fragrance of fresh produce and coffee, not like today's convenience stores with their sterile, impersonal atmosphere or sprawling supermarkets with their ubiquitous generic piped-in music, steroid-and-red-dye-injected, cellophane-encased, antiseptic beef-steak and disengaged check-out girls and sackboys, their brains gone slack from the ceaseless chirp of the comput-erized price-tag scanner. "Paper or plastic?" "You have a work phone?" "Have a nice day!"

My grandfather had a lifelong affection for grocery stores and grocers. (My mother never went grocery shop-ping with us and, as far as I know, never went at all until I started taking her with me after Raymond died.) Crow Grocery on Cleburne's east side was nearest to our house on English Street and the one we went to most often. But across the Henderson Street bridge, going toward town, was Burd's Grocery, a more general operation than Crow's, not only in name but in merchandise as well. Several miles to the south, across from Adams Elementary School, was Givens' Grocery, owned and operated by R.E. Givens and his son, Charles. On the way to Givens' store we would walk past Burd's Grocery, Parkway, Dempwolf's, Wofford's, Wiggins', Cash Service, Ball's, and Safeway. We walked to Givens' store at least once a month, passing up all these nearer stores, most of them with a much greater variety of items. Either Mr. Givens or Charles would bring us home in a car with our groceries. My grandfather did this because, during the Depression, Mr. Givens let him have groceries on credit when he didn't have the money to pay. For several years he couldn't pay a penny on his bill. Then, when he got a job moving houses, he began paying him back. My grandfather told me that you don't forget a kindness like that. "I could buy groceries cheaper at Safeway," he said, "but if I ever got to where I couldn't pay, I'd be stuck. Elgie Givens let me have the groceries and never asked me for a dime."

Sometimes, on Saturday nights, we stopped at Burd's on the way back home from town and bought groceries. It was a neighborhood store, similar in size to Givens' but more boisterous. Ted Burd, a chunky, intense man with an ever-present cigar stub in his mouth, always seemed to be hurrying up and down the aisles, from his office at the front of the store to the meat market and back again. His office had a roll-top desk piled high with paperwork, and a large framed picture of Franklin Roosevelt hung on the wall. The meat department was loud and frenzied, as the butcher, Bill Randolph, barked orders to his assistant, Pee Wee, who was also his brother, and to the stock boy, Bill Miller. This one-man rendering plant wore a white cap and apron and puffed maniacally on a cigar stub. Ashes floated down into the meat as he chopped and sawed and sliced and hammered with his crooked, arthritic hands, sweat coursing down his forehead from beneath his white paper hat. Meat spatterings dribbling off his chin mixed with the sweat and ashes to season the packinghouse-fresh, non-steroid-and-non-red-dye-injected, butcher-paper-wrapped-and-twine-tied USDA grade-A roasts and steaks.

My favorite store was Crow Grocery, owned and operated by brothers Burnice and Charley "Shorty" Crow. Burnice, a pleasant pie-faced man with dry, serpentine skin who always wore loose Williamson-Dickie khakis and short-sleeved sport shirts, sketched portraits of movie stars and presidents and clipped them to a wire across the store with clothespins. I always looked to make sure Marilyn and Ava were still there, then, if I had a nickel, I went to the cold drink box and fished a Mission Orange out of the almost unbearably cold water. Coconut Snowballs, chocolate cream-filled cupcakes, Devil Dogs, fried pies, cinnamon rolls, and every other sweet morsel you could imagine lined the racks. Next to this was the candy case, dozens of colorfully wrapped bars lined up in neat rows like platoons of glossy soldiers in full-dress parade formation. Burnice called me "Bosko." I never knew why. He used to say, "Bosko just eats once a day—from the time he gets up till the time he goes to bed." His brother, "Shorty," was almost blind and walked by holding to countertops and furniture and swinging his body along on truncated, misshapen legs. My grandmother said their parents were cousins.

I was her errand boy during the day when she needed something on short notice, but my favorite time to go was in the evening with my grandfather when he went up there for his Prince Albert and to socialize with his friends from the neighborhood. My grandfather was a humble and uneducated farmer, tall and slender with a bald dome as brown as pork roast and a tint of red on the back of the neck. He had blue eyes and huge nurturing hands and fingers that looked like big brown cucumbers. I've never seen anyone hold a baby as tenderly as he did. Children went to sleep in his arms as if they were sedated. Those magnificent weather-beaten hands caressed them and patted their bottoms in a lulling, rhythmic cadence that sent them into almost instant comforting, dream-filled sleep. "By-yo baby," he would say over and over as he patted. Inside my mother's old trunk there is a fading photo of him in his overalls and hat, sitting on the wooden steps of our house on James Street, holding me, still an infant, in his arms, with happiness shining in my face like Karo syrup.

His hair was gone on top by the time I came along, but he used to brush his head with the clothes brush. Before we got a bathroom, he took baths in the summertime under the hackberry tree in the backyard in a washtub. The neighbors were used to it, I guess. Then he'd shave before the mirror in his bedroom, splash on lots of Old Spice and smell like a million bucks. After he did all that, his face seemed to shine like one of my grandmother's kitchen pans.

He met his friends up at "Shorty's" most evenings after supper to talk and smoke and listen to *Amos 'n' Andy* and *Lum and Abner*. Mr. Alexander, a big fat friendly man in overalls who lived across the street from the store, always got the broom and swept the wooden floor as he talked. My grandfather said it was because his wife made him do it so much at home that he couldn't talk without sweeping. Every now and then a customer would drive into the driveway and Shorty would hobble out and pump gas out of one of those old-time manually operated pumps.

The men stood around and smoked Prince Albert and leaned on the counter and talked of the old days. Their talk centered on farming, though they all had given up that life and now worked for the railroad. They talked about how hard the Depression had been, friends who had died, and other real things they had a part in. There was no talk of sports or movies or gossip. The only celebrity they knew or cared about, other than Roy Acuff, Red Foley, or a few other *Grand Ole Opry* performers, was Mr. Roosevelt, called "Ruzyvelt." Sometimes, one would say that he had to roof his house tomorrow, set up a fence, or some other such chore and, after work, the others would show up with their tools, to help get the job done. These images returned to me over the years for a long time after that when I smelled the aroma of Prince Albert. I even went through a period of smoking it myself when I worked for the railroad. My grandfather eventually gave it up when Dr. Cooke had to remove a cancer from his lip.

My grandfather and I never missed a Joe Louis fight on radio. For the Louis–Charles fight in 1950, I talked him into walking to Dickson's Furniture Store and watching it on television, hoping he would get interested in buying one. He said he'd think about it. Two years later, in time for the Democratic National Convention, he bought a twelve-inch Zenith with a tinted screen that gave the illusion of color. When the scene was just right, such as in a western when the action was outdoors, you had green vegetation and blue sky. More often, though, as in the convention shots, you got politicians with green clothes and blue faces.

We used to watch Adlai Stevenson's speeches in their entirety, and I wasn't allowed to talk or make noise while they were on. Back then, presidential candidates made long speeches outlining their proposals, sometimes lasting for an hour or more. Stevenson's were brilliant, insightful, witty, punctuated with literary and biblical allusions — and self-written. "I will not talk down to the American people," he said, and lost to Eisenhower by a landslide. That year, I had begun associating at school with the "rich" kids from the other side of town and, when our civics teacher gave us the assignment to make a campaign speech for our candidate, I noticed that most of them supported Eisenhower. The only time my grandfather ever threatened to whip me was the time I came home from school and said that maybe Eisenhower wouldn't make such a bad president.

Summer nights my mother and I sometimes walked across town to the city park to watch the softball games. This was several years before Little League came to Cleburne. On Saturday nights all the stores were open downtown, and a boy could break away from his mother long enough to rush into Brown-Bilt shoe store and see his footbones in the x-ray machine. On hot nights, the stores had their doors open, and the town was rich with things to see and smell. The flavorful aroma of the produce and coffee greeted you a long way before you got to the grocery stores. After we crossed South Main Street at the Grandview Highway, I started smelling the chlorine from the city pool, the park's centerpiece, which my grandfather helped build when he worked for the Works Progress Administration for a dollar a day. We sat in the limestone stands, also built by the WPA, and I marveled at these local heroes struggling on the field. Though they were hardly more than teenagers themselves, they were like demigods to me, especially the pitchers. It was fast-pitch in those days, and some of them could really burn it in there. The best there ever was, say most of the players still living, was Red Norman. He had a specialty pitch called a "slow rise ball" that almost always caught batters off guard after a fastball. The Stepp brothers, the boys who lived in the house across the street from us when I cut my thumb off, were pitcher and catcher for King Brothers, one of the best teams. Cecil, the catcher, died in a car crash in the spring of 1965. The other, W. F. "Dub," married my wife's aunt. In a small town, it seems that everything is connected in some way.

Another star player, Bill Burleson, who played for the Dillon Hot Shots (an odd name for a team representing a funeral home), married the grown sister of a playmate of mine who lived two doors down on English Street. They went on a fishing trip with her brother, "Jonesy," and his wife. A storm came up and overturned their boat. Jonesy rescued his sister, but his wife and brother-in-law drowned. This was the saddest thing I remember from our neighborhood. I always thought it was odd that he would save his sister over his wife, but biogeneticists nowadays would say that he was subconsciously saving himself because he shared genes with his sister and none with his wife or brother-in-law.

My love of baseball extended to the minor leagues. Evenings when my mother was out on dates with Raymond, I tuned in the Fort Worth Cats games from La Grave Field, announced by Bill Hightower. They had some great players in those days who went on to star in the big leagues. Duke Snider was probably the most famous, but also there were Chico Carresquel, Dee Fondy, Bobby Bragan, Carl Erskine, Carl Spooner, and Don Hoak. On one occasion, they brought in Chico's family from Venezuela and landed on the field in something unimaginable to me called a helicopter. They did this because he was homesick for them, and the owners didn't want to take the chance that their star shortstop might go into a slump.

One evening in late spring, an old panel truck was seen parked across the road behind our house, alongside Buffalo Creek. It had "The Incredible Aeolus, the Human Bellows" written on the side in large letters. A couple of my friends and I went down there to investigate. An old man sat on the running board of the vehicle. He wore a pair of khaki shorts with no shirt or shoes. His skin was like leather and dark as a smoked turkey. A network of tendons crisscrossed his chest. His arms and legs were thin, and he looked like a bullfrog because he had a big barrel chest. I was thoughtlessly pulling up grass by the roots as he talked to us about the sights of the world he had seen. He looked at me and said gently: "The grass is food for livestock, son, and some people use it for a roof over their heads. We must preserve growing things and they will preserve us." He seemed very old to us then, about a hundred, but he might not have been over fifty. We were about ten years old.

He showed us how he could suck in his stomach all the way to his backbone. Then, the Human Bellows picked up an inner tube for a truck tire lying beside him and began blowing into it. It began to expand. Up... up... up... until we thought it would explode. A vein protruded on his forehead. The tube swelled with his breath until it was higher than the fender of the car. He stopped, the vein on his forehead pulsating. His bulging eyes shone like agates. "Never smoke cigarettes," he told us, "and don't waste your breath on opinions, promises, excuses, or sermons. Save your breath," he added, "and your breath will save you." He spoke in these palindromes and seemed ever so much more profound than anyone I had ever heard before. I thought of the old man a dozen years later when I heard President Kennedy, a fancier of palindromes, say, "Ask not what your country can do for you but what you can do for your country." Had "the Amazing Aeolus, the Human Bellows" taken his show to the schoolchildren of Massachusetts?

The next day our teacher took us down to the small stage in the cafeteria where we saw the same old man blow up inner tubes for the whole school. Then he told the children the same thing he told us on the creek bank. We couldn't stop telling everybody how we had a private show the day before. For a while after that, we all had to have bicycle inner tubes to blow up. "Look at me! I'm the Amazing Aeolus!" became a familiar neighborhood cry. We soon tired of this fantasy, though, and went back to our usual games, and I eventually violated all of the old man's teachings. But it was the best thing I ever learned in school.

Soon after I became a teacher, I learned that these wonders of our childhood stood for little with this new generation of students who had seen thousands of miraculous feats in the cool, detached images of television's daily light; an old man who could suck his stomach all the way in to his backbone and stick pins into his skin and blow up the inner tube of a truck tire with his breath was but dross compared to the daily feast of wonders at their disposal. By the light of its flickering magic, television made an instant anachronism of my vision of the world based on small wonders like neighborhood grocery stores and the Milky Way and slingshots and marbles and mustang grapes, and rendered my values as obsolete as the anatomical talents of an old swami and his palindromatic teachings.

Had I stopped to think about it, I would have wanted that life forever but, in time, the Captain Midnight De-Coder rings and marbles were replaced by cars and beer and girls in hoop skirts who became wives, and suddenly the ones who would be kids forever had kids of their own and paid rent on row houses with air conditioners and televisions instead of wide gossipy front porches that caught the breeze from the cool wet lawns of a faraway small-town yesterday.

CHAPTER
SIX

D addy was good at building
a fire in the fireplace. We used to start out by sitting way back
from it, then move closer and closer to it as it died out. When
it went out, we went to bed. Coon, that silly thing, used to
wait till we all got in bed, then go outside and pretend he was
bringing in wood. He'd bang on the front door and holler till
one of us would get up out of our warm bed and go open the
door for him. "Somebody come out here and open this door for
me! I'm freezing!" When we did, he'd be just standing there,
not a stick of wood in his hand. He'd turn his hands over to
show us he didn't have any wood, then laugh like a hyena. I
could have killed him.

He was Daddy's pet, I think. While we were hoeing, he got
to ride on the plow. And when he got old enough, Daddy let

him do the plowing. He liked to do that because it was easier than hoeing. Daddy was particular about everything, and me and Bernice couldn't suit him in the field like Coon and Wayne could. But she turned out to be just like him. If she was a man she'd be Daddy made over. Coon and Bernice look alike and me and Wayne favor.

Daddy went to town every Saturday and Mama would let me and Bernice ride the horse while he was gone. He always took Coon and Wayne with him because they were boys. He'd bring us a stick of candy, but he'd have used a switch on us if he'd ever found out we were riding the horse while he was gone. It was Daddy's favorite horse. It was blind. He said it came off the racetrack.

Coon's real name is W. L. but Mama and Daddy were the only ones that called him that. Everybody else calls him Coon. I think they started calling him Coon because he always had an old coon dog with him everywhere he went. He was always acting silly and getting in trouble at school. He acted like that up to the time that your cousin Durwood got hit in the head by a flying Coke bottle and died. He changed after that. But he was a real nut. One time he was acting a fool and playing like he had the Holy Ghost. He had been to a Holy Roller tent meeting down on East Henderson and came home and started acting like he was imitating them. He put one of Mama's cro-cheted doilies on top of his head and started shaking and acting a fool, and the next thing we knew he had her crochet needle stuck in the palm of his hand. Mama said it was because he was making fun of the Holy Rollers.

Growing up on English Street, I learned about the man who was said to be my father because I sometimes over-heard my mother talking about him to the other women she worked with at Woolworth's and because he sent letters and packages with lots of interesting oddities and goodies in them, like Nazi medals and photos of German soldiers he said he shot. There would be an X marked on the picture to show where the bullet had hit the enemy soldier. I slipped around and looked through these treasures when she was working.

I even saw him once, when he came to our house with his army uniform on in the middle of the night. I was about five years old. He stayed a few days. He walked with me down to the creek behind our house, and one night they took me swimming at the city park. I stayed in the baby pool because I hadn't learned how to swim. "Look at me!" I remember yelling to them. "Watch me swim!" I was just crawling around on the bottom. Even then I was skilled in fantasy.

He brought with him a wooden box filled with a trove of captured booty. He left it with us and I looked at the treasures in the box over and over for a long time. There were gold pocket watches with precious gems on the dial, pearl necklaces, women's wristwatches and gold necklaces, two leather pouches of straight razors, leather trousers, a Luger pistol, a couple of daggers, a swastika medal, several Nazi stickpins and, oddly, some pornographic photographs. Now, only three razors are left, a necklace or two, a decorative shaving mug, a beaded mosaic place mat, and the wooden box they came in. Everything else has disappeared. I always suspected that my mother sold it all to Fay Burton, one of the local jewelers. The leather pants stayed outside in the back yard and got stiff from the rain and sun. In a drawer of the desk I am writing on, I have his letters to me, some of his personal effects, his Bronze Star, a Purple Heart, a Combat

Infantryman's Badge, and several campaign ribbons. His sister, my Aunt Edith, gave them to me after he died.

When he came in that night, Aunt Bernice had gone to the door and, thinking she was my mother, he kissed her by mistake. When he finally learned the difference between the sisters, he went to bed with us and got on top of my mother. "This is the first I've had since I was in France," I heard him say. My mother had felt of my eyelids in some sort of foolish attempt to see if I was asleep. I simply closed my eyes. The bed began to shake. Aunt Bernice was lucky she missed out on this, I thought.

He gave me a pearl-handled pocketknife the next day and left. I still have the knife. On one handle he had scratched, "A. B. Dodge," and on the other, "Tommie." I never saw him again and, of course, he was never mentioned to me by anyone in the household. It is like a dream. If it weren't for the knife, I would wonder whether it really happened at all.

Then Raymond started showing up in front of our house in his light blue 1937 Plymouth. He didn't honk his horn, just stopped in front and she went out. He had a narrow waist, slender hips, and wide shoulders, one of which he carried lower than the other. He always wore a fedora back then, and I thought he looked like Randolph Scott. Typically, there was no explanation from her of who he was and why she was leaving with him. Aunt Bernice finally told me; otherwise I would have had to figure it out for myself. I used to put nails in the street in front of our house to make him have a flat, but this strategy brought little success, as he kept coming.

In 1952, when I was thirteen, they stayed out all night. The next morning they told my grandparents they had gotten married. No one ever said anything to me about it.

"If they can make a go of it," said my grandfather over breakfast, "it's all right with me."

My grandmother didn't say anything for a long time. Then, she said, "If she can live with him, I can live by him."

He took her to live in Pampa, a town in far west Texas about the same size as Cleburne, and I stayed with my grandparents. I was angry with her for going away with this man I didn't like and leaving me without a word of explanation.

That's when I started getting into trouble at school.

I began playing hooky a lot, with the boys from the other side of town, the "nice" side of the tracks. This was in the seventh grade. Bad grades began showing up on my report cards. A reputation as a troublemaker wasn't far behind, and teachers stopped being friendly to me. At Santa Fe Elementary, my teachers had taken me to other classes to read and recite for the children in the upper classes. I was always a favorite of the elementary teachers because I could read without moving my lips.

I was also a favorite of the principal. During this time an incident occurred that, were it to happen today to a schoolchild, would have very different results. Our principal was an exemplary educator and family man. He was always impeccably dressed in a double-breasted suit and fedora. He was a faithful supporter of the Cleburne Yellow Jackets football team and went to all the games, at home and away. It was a great honor to be asked, along with the other boys, to go with him in his new 1949 De Soto on the trips out of town to see the games. Other than through my books and radio, these trips were my only contact with the world outside Cleburne. We went to faraway places like Irving, Dallas, Graham, Breckenridge, and Brownwood.

It was also a great honor to be chosen to push the button in his office and ring the school bell that changed classes and ended the school day. A lot of times, he would tell me what a smart and wonderful boy I was and give me a big kiss. These weren't little pecks on the cheek. They were big manly smackers that smashed my mouth almost all the way around to my ear. I also viewed these kisses from the principal as a high honor. I had seen pictures in the *National Geographic* of men in other countries kissing each other and thought he must be from one of these countries. Kisses were as far as it went, but today, just these kisses would cost him his job, his reputation, and maybe his marriage. Looking back on my own such incident, I consider it the only demonstration of affection I ever received from an adult.

When I got to junior high it all changed. The teachers and principals whacked me with a board instead of kissing me and, instead of attention, I was given detention and suspension. I assumed the punishment was a result of my growing proclivity for sarcasm and wisecracks in my answers to teachers' questions. Examples of my considerably less-than-erudite humor:

"Tommy, which country have you selected to report on?"

"I'll take the Virgin Islands."

And this certain detonator of laughter that got me in trouble with a literature teacher:

"Tommy, what did Brutus do to Caesar that caused Caesar to say, 'Et tu, Brute'?"

"Uh, he said, 'How many eggs did you eat for breakfast this morning, Caesar?'"

This kind of thing.

Soon after I became a teacher, I learned that teachers

often form judgments about children by the way they look and by the clothes they wear. I probably didn't present too promising a figure as a student in my homemade clothes and carrying my sandwich in a Mrs. Baird's bread sack. Among these affluent and "culturally enrichened" children, I must have looked like Huckleberry Finn at Harvard. I might have come out of it, though, if some teacher had just put her arm around me and told me how well I could read and recite. I wasn't "bad," but I wanted the same attention I had in elementary school. The punishment added to my pain, but at least I wasn't ignored. Punishment never makes anyone a better person, but it does bring recognition.

I was, though, still capable of making good grades, probably because I read so much. In addition to comic books, baseball record books and the like, I read lots of history and biography. I also became, at an early age, interested in famous lawyers and celebrated trials of the past. My courtroom hero wasn't Perry Mason. I liked Clarence Darrow. At twelve, when my friends were taking their first awkward steps toward the dance floor with girls, I had gleaned every detail of the Leopold-Loeb trial from the library's back issues of the *Cleburne Times Review*. It was comforting to me that you could do something as horribly wrong as kidnap and murder a child and still have someone defend you. If a case could be made to defend those two boys, then certainly there was hope for me. I wished that Clarence Darrow was my father.

It was about this time that something happened in Cleburne that absorbed a good deal of my attention for months. A good-looking nineteen-year-old boy named Arthur Clayton Hester was put on trial in the Johnson County courthouse for the murder of Dr. John Lord, a history professor at Texas Christian University. I tried to get my mother to take me to the trial, but she wouldn't do it because it involved S-E-X. If she wouldn't even allow me to go see a movie called *The Naked City*, she certainly wasn't going to allow me to attend a murder trial involving a kind of sex "that dares not speak its name," as homosexuality was identified in the press in those days. So, instead of going to the trial I had to make do by reading every sanitized word of the proceedings in the newspaper.

Hester was an impoverished boy who had lived with his mother in a dirt-floor hovel in Fort Worth when he met Dr. Lord in a movie theater. The professor moved him into his Johnson County farmhouse and clothed and educated him. Trouble started when the boy asked to borrow the professor's car to take a girl on a date. There was an argument and a fight, in which Hester killed the professor with an iron pipe. Instead of driving his girl on a date, he fled in the car to his sister's house in California. He was arrested there and returned to the Johnson County jail for trial.

He was a stunningly handsome boy, and the Cleburne girls all wanted to see him in person. He looked like James Dean, who came along four or five years later. Hester was convicted in 18th District Court and received a fifty-year sentence. He was released after ten years and got a job in Dallas driving a truck. Today, by using the defense that he had been sexually abused by the professor, he might have been acquitted.

My grandfather wasn't one of his admirers. One day, when we were down at the lumberyard, located directly behind the jail, we heard someone yell at us from one of the jail windows. He said, "Hey, old man, why don't you come up and get my autograph! I'm Arthur Clayton Hester!"

I couldn't believe it. My eyes must have bugged out on stems. My grandfather hardly looked up. In his reply he used a word I had never heard him use before. He said: "Naw. I've seen queers before."

My brewing troubles in school boiled over one morning in crafts class. One of my favorite teachers, Mr. Anderson, a jovial and befreckled Henry the Eighth look-alike, asked me to desist hammering while he talked. I kept on. "If you hammer one more time," he warned, "you're going to the office."

Of course, I hammered one more time.

The principal, Mr. Jackson, a soft-spoken man with feline features, told me what the punishment would be.

I had made up my mind there would be no more whippings.

"Either take the licks or you're expelled."

I walked out of his office and went home. The next day I had a bus ticket to Pampa.

CHAPTER
SEVEN

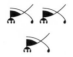

You always liked to go around
the boys that treated you the worst. The meaner they were to
you the better you liked them. When you were in high school I
couldn't make you stop hanging around with those older boys
down at that shoe shop across from the square. They used to
gamble down there and you'd be right in the middle of all of it.
They were too old for you but nothing could stop you. You just
loved them.

When you were just a little boy you used to love to play with
Darrell Walker and he'd do mean things to you. Next day,
back you'd go. He'd hit you or hold you down and choke you
and take your funny books away from you and you'd come
home crying. But you liked him. You always liked the older
boys and the ones that got in trouble. He used to pick on you

and got you to smoking cigarettes. You never liked the ones that went to Sunday school and church. The meaner they were the better you liked them. Darrell grew up to be a good man, though. I never thought he would.

I was too young to realize it then, but I wasn't wanted in Pampa, either. My mother lived with Raymond in a one-bedroom apartment and made no plans to move to a bigger place when I arrived. Their apartment was attached to the house at 706 North West Street owned by Mr. and Mrs. Cloud Drew. Mrs. Drew was a kind but ceaselessly chattering society matron, arrayed morning to night in the kind of sartorial finery reserved in our household for Sundays or funerals. When she learned that I was a budding sportswriter, she said that she had seen but one football game in her life and that it had been a disappointment. "A player," she said, "sailed the ball between his legs to another boy, who kicked it out of the stadium and I never saw it again." Mr. Drew was a portly, dough-faced man of middle-class means, the owner of a plumbing supply business. He liked opera, and I remember trying to go to sleep with the unrelenting voice of Blanche Thebom penetrating the walls. I slept on a cot in the tiny kitchen. I believe this early experience with opera explains to this day my stubborn antipathy toward this particular form of entertainment and the zeal with which I peruse the obituary section of the newspaper each day, looking for the name of a mezzo soprano.

I don't recall much about our home life in that two-room apartment except that Raymond didn't speak to me during this time or, for that matter, for about five years after he and my mother got married.

I made good grades in that school, but it was a strange, even eerie, experience, being with classmates who had started in the first grade together and knew each other as well as I knew my friends at home. I felt terribly alone but made two friends: Tommy Vehon and Bill Gurley. They smoked cigarettes and had their own Ronson lighters. Tommy was a stocky boy with swarthy features, protruding forehead, and looked, I thought, like a diminutive Max Schmeling, the German boxer who fought Joe Louis on behalf of the Aryan race. Bill was red-headed and ruddy, with a hearty, Irish laugh. To me they were the Dead-End Kids of the Texas Panhandle. There's no question that they were the nonpareils of the pool table. They taught me to play and took me to the Pampa Coney Island Cafe for the first time. We played pool after school at the Clover Club, a Dickensian region at the top of a dark stairway where old men with garters on their sleeves and pee stains on their pants sat and smoked and played dominoes underneath a hanging hooded light. A withered man wearing a green visor and immersed in smoke sat on a stool in a small caged room at the top of the stairs. He took your money mechanically and went back to reading *Police Gazette*. Some afternoons, a couple of roughnecks from the oil fields would come in, and they would drink from a pint of whiskey hidden in their jackets. To a boy from Cleburne, where pool halls were outlawed and whiskey was illegal, iniquity hung in the air like a fetid nicotine cloud.

Bill and Tommy, these two friendly wastrels, treated me better than my friends at home did. I learned many years later that when a new person comes in, it is always the alienated ones who befriend him first.

My teacher was Mrs. Rankin, a beautiful woman with a

complexion the color of piano keys and shining black hair pulled back and tied tightly behind her head. She read Tennyson's "Enoch Arden" to us in its entirety. I was interested in Enoch. He was also separated from his family and friends.

In the evenings, sometimes Mr. and Mrs. Drew invited us to watch television with them. Liberace was their favorite. After a few times of this, I stayed in the apartment and listened to the Pampa Harvesters' basketball games on the radio. They had a great high school team and won the state championship several seasons in a row. They had a center named Jimmy Bond who was six-five and could dunk the ball, an unheard-of feat in those days, certainly among high school players. The other players were Gary Griffin, E. J. McIlvain, Harold Lewis, and Ken Hinkle. I added these to my growing list of heroes. Griffin and McIlvain became star players at Rice and Hinkle at North Texas State College, now the University of North Texas. I don't know what happened to Jimmy Bond. I heard he became a preacher, I guess to slam-dunk Satan through the basketball hoop of life.

I finished out the semester there and went back home to Cleburne. Raymond took me to the bus station and gave me ten dollars. "Here!" he said, holding out the bill for me to take.

"Thanks," I said.

This was memorable because we ordinarily didn't have conversations.

But trouble was waiting in Cleburne, and I returned to my old habits of playing hooky and making bad grades. In the fall semester of 1953, I left that school again. I went back to the small apartment and sleeping on the cot, to Bill Gurley, the Pampa Coney Island Cafe, and the

Clover Club. In Cleburne, my reputation had hurt me with the football coaches, and my athletic career came to an end in the ninth grade. Most of the coaches viewed me as a troublemaker and a "wise guy." In a game I took a hard smash to the hip bone and had to be carried to the sidelines. Dr. Yater, who became my grandfather's doctor after Dr. Cooke died, was in the stands. He drove me home in his Cadillac, with my bike in the trunk. I told myself this injury was the reason I didn't make the team, but the real reason was that I was too small, too fat, and too distracted to compete with the other boys. In Pampa I didn't even try.

But I wanted my friends in Cleburne to believe that I was a star player at my new school. I managed to get a Reaper letter, a white "P" for Pampa, from one of my pool hall friends and sewed it onto a blue sweater my mother bought for me. It looked authentic. My Cleburne friends would be jealous because they had only a letter and no sweater, and the coaches would be sorry they hadn't known how to make better use of my great athletic ability. The hoax didn't work, however, and everybody learned that my talent was for fantasy, not football. A classmate, a star player, simply looked inside the pocket and said, "Where's your name?" I hadn't known that the player's name is always sewed inside the lining of the pocket.

In Pampa, I made another friend this time, a wiry, dark-haired boy by the name of Kelly Davis. He was older than his classmates and had a tough-guy reputation despite his down-sized physique. The word went out one day that he was going to fight Burl Kirby at the Red Brick, our cafeteria building, at lunch period. Burl, a star lineman on the Reapers football team, was six inches taller and about forty pounds heavier than Kelly. I've always been interested in names and their power, especially unconscious power, over the person associated with them—that a boy who grew up on English Street would become an English teacher, for example. Would Mr. Givens have been so benevolent to his grocery customers if he had been Mr. Buckholder? And would Burl still have grown up "burly" if his parents had named him Percy? My Uncle Wayne always called me "Oscar Wilde" when I was growing up. I'm glad I didn't know until I went to college who my namesake was, otherwise I might have grown up liking cucumber sandwiches and flute recitals instead of chili dogs and boxing. In this particular match, I feared the worst but was there at Kelly's side, urging him on. It was snowing and very cold. The fighters wore gloves—not boxing gloves, just ordinary leather gloves—to keep their fists from freezing in the frigid air. Burl said, "I'll let you have the first punch." Kelly punched him with everything he had, but Burl shrugged it off as he would a pesky mosquito and then broke Kelly's collar bone with one punch. That, of course, ended the fight.

I went to see my hero in the hospital. He looked like a sick, frightened child. It wouldn't be the last time I would see a hero deflated.

Four years later as a freshman at North Texas State College, I ran into Burl Kirby. "Hi, Burl," I said, "remember me?"

He looked me over and seemed to make an attempt at what is known as a normal recollection. "No," he said. "Who are you?"

"Your guess is as good as mine," I said and went on my way, disappointed but not surprised that yet another person failed to verify my identity. Someone born with a blank birth certificate can't ever get enough verification.

I never ate at the Red Brick. Every day I ran at top speed downtown to the Coney Island Cafe, where you could get wonderful coneys for ten cents each with lots of cheese and onions and chili, a Coke for a nickel, and a slice of homemade pie for fifteen cents. Two brothers ran the place, dishing up these treats to crashing throngs of hungry students, businessmen, city officials in suits and, at one time or another, just about everybody in the county.

In 1985, on the way to New Mexico, I took Brenda through Pampa to show her all my old memories. Mrs. Drew was still there, though Cloud had gone on to that great plumbing supply warehouse in the sky. My old school was torn down, and I had a hard time remembering where it had been. What would the Pampa Coney Island Cafe be now? A video store probably, I said.

We parked on the street across from the courthouse, and I saw Tarpley's music store where my mother bought my first guitar and told the saleslady that I didn't have any musical ability. I guess she was right. I never learned a single chord until a boy in my barracks at Fort Jackson, North Carolina, taught me A, G, and E. After that, I was guilty of playing a few unrecognizable tunes.

Down the street, Addington's Western Store was still standing, where she had bought me a large maroon cowboy hat. Back in Cleburne, later, a friend's father said, "That's a big hat for such a little squirt." I sold it after that, on the installment plan, to an older boy for $10.

Turning the corner onto West Foster Street I told Brenda, "It won't be there, but I can show you where it used to be."

Oh, my lord, the Coney Island Cafe was still there! After all these years! I wondered who owned the place now. Probably some mom-and-pop team from Muskogee who had given up the Amway dealership. No, it was the same two brothers, John and Ted Geikas, still heating up the coneys on the same grill in the front window! I gazed at the same Naugahyde and chrome-trimmed booths, the same stools lined up beside the same counter. I was greatly moved by the sights and smells of something so pleasant from an otherwise unhappy period. It's a wonderful thing to see something from your childhood remain unchanged. It's saddening to me to see office buildings and the like going up virtually overnight where old and familiar landmarks used to be. Developers cement over our childhoods and brick up our memories. Executives transact business deals on the spot where we transacted romantic business in the back seat of a first car.

I gorged myself on memory. I ordered two coneys, a Coke, and a slice of coconut pie from one of the seventeen pies that John had made that morning, as he does every morning of his life except Sundays. For holidays, he makes forty-five. The coneys were eighty cents now, still a bargain, the Coke a quarter, and the pie eighty cents. It all tasted exactly the same. It was still served on glass plates, the drinks in real glasses, no Styrofoam, no plastic. I looked toward the door, half-expecting to see Jimmy Bond and the rest of the glorious Harvesters come bounding in.

I told John that I had come back after thirty years to eat these same coneys. He called his brother over, and we all chatted for a few minutes. They told me a remarkable story. The cafe, John said, was twenty years old when I used to eat there as a child. Their uncle started it in 1933, and they bought it from him after World War II. It hasn't changed except for the refrigeration system. He said Bob Wills used to wash dishes for them, and Woody Guthrie, a close friend of John's, used to hang around there. John said Woody wrote a song about the place called "All Alone on Saturday Night." Later, I searched for the record for several months, even wrote to folksinger Pete Seeger, who didn't know it but told me to check with the Woody Guthrie Foundation, where I also drew a blank. John still maintains the story is true. It doesn't matter. The Coney Island Cafe is one of the best memories I have of that town.

But leaving Cleburne didn't solve my behavior problems. There were times when I fell back into my old ways. One of the worst was the trouble I got into in shop class. The teacher was Mr. Ritter, and naturally everybody called him "Tex" behind his back. I didn't realize nobody called him that to his face, until I did it one day. Furiously angry, he sent me out of the class and told me to stay out. That weekend I went up to the school and did something shameful. I took some chalk and wrote "Tex is a queer" on the sidewalk in front of his shop classroom. I didn't know what that word meant exactly but had heard my grandfather use it disdainfully that day in the lumberyard. I thought it meant something similar to a "freak." The other boys had a saying: "I'd rather be a freak for a week than a queer for a year." As I remember it, the ambiguity of the rhyme left a question in my mind as to which epithet carried more derision. After considerable analysis I settled on the latter as having more heft as an insult.

I never went back to that school. For a few days I hung out at the pool hall instead of going to class. I felt that I didn't fit in anywhere. Then I told my mother I was going back to Cleburne. She never knew I had a problem in the world.

She had her own problems. She cried all the time to go back home.

CHAPTER EIGHT

W hen I was born, Daddy
had the typhoid fever and the doctor told Mama he was probably going to die. She had to get a nurse because I was a baby
and had to hire hands to get in the crop. She had to cook for
them and carry water too. We didn't have a well. That was in
February of 1918. The baby had just died and Uncle Dock
had just left for the service and all that really got Mama down.
Her and Uncle Dock hadn't ever been separated before and it
like to have killed her. She said she was afraid she'd never see
him again. He wrote us lots of letters. The last one he wrote
was from France. We were told a shell exploded and killed
him. It happened a few days after he wrote the letter. But we
never knew for sure how it really happened. Grandma James
lost her mind over it. He was a good boy. Mama talked about

*him till the day she died. She always said how much he liked
school. And he was good to take care of Coon. He would even
go along with Daddy when he went to town and look after
Coon and even change his diapers. He was studying to make
a preacher. We heard about Uncle Dock all our lives.*

My mother's family history was one of profound adver-
sity. I remember the times my grandmother read to me
from the Book of Job, her favorite Bible story. I never
brought it up to her but, even as a child, I was bothered by
the fact that Job was tortured because of a kind of celestial
argument between God and Satan. The idea was that God
would prove Satan wrong when he contended that no
man would remain faithful to God if enough torture were
applied. So, God sends this humble farmer financial ruin
and inflamed boils, then kills all his children. Personally,
I didn't like the implication that these two competing
deities might also be using my mother—and me—as
experiments in some kind of cosmic laboratory.

Eventually, from her stories and from rummaging
through the old trunk, I learned all about the tragedies of
her life. My mother's disease would have been just one
more burden for my grandmother to bear. She would have
known it much earlier than I did and handled it a lot better, too. She would have detected it despite my mother's
cleverness at covering it up.

One of my mother's tactics was stonewalling and
diverting in the face of direct questions, usually waiting
for Raymond to come to the rescue. If he didn't, she
improvised. Question: "Did you work today?" Answer:
"Uh, I'm so tired of that job I don't know what to do.
Sometimes my back just kills me after lifting those kids."

When she didn't know the answer to a question like "Have you seen Lindon today?" she would simply mumble something unintelligible and repair to the kitchen to start frying biscuits. When she initiated a conversation, it was always about the past. When Raymond's tight-lippedness is factored in, it is more understandable that her condition came as such a surprise to me. He came from the old school that viewed mental illness as a disgrace. He used to say that so-and-so "went off," in a kind of whisper that indicated it wasn't something you said out loud.

I should have known in January of 1991 when I did a Gulf War-related radio commentary on Uncle Dock. Though she had never listened to any of my commentaries, I thought she would want to hear this one. I told her all about it, the times it would air and so forth, and set her radio on KERA the night before. Before I went to bed I called her and asked her to turn her radio on so that I could be sure it was still on the station. It was.

The next day I drove down to see them. "Did you listen to me on the radio talking about Uncle Dock?" I said.

That look of panic and confusion, so familiar to me now, flashed across her face. Raymond went about his tinkering, saying nothing. "I count on Raymond to —" she said, obviously flustered. "To remind me of everything" was what she was going to say before she stopped herself. He never said one word. I guess I wasn't particularly alarmed because she had never shown any interest in my doings before. I shrugged it off.

On his eightieth birthday, Raymond said, "This will be my last birthday." Eleven months later, minus two days, he died.

For the last five years before I retired, I stopped teaching on Fridays and used that day to go to Cleburne. For some reason, on that last Friday of his life, I didn't go but called him on the phone. We talked for a long time about Lowell's new truck and how he needed to go down and buy one for himself—a long conversation—but, characteristically, he didn't mention that he was deathly ill. I knew he going downhill but, other than urge the children to visit him more often, I tried to block it out. He had stopped smoking five years before, but the effects over sixty years of it had left him wrinkled and drawn, weak and unable to breathe without that rattling sound. What I perceived in the two of them was like something from a Thomas Hardy novel: his perfect brain in a wasted body; her youthful, perfect body and a deteriorating brain.

The next day, I went down there around noon. They were sitting at the table, eating hamburgers. Every day he went and bought something for lunch. (Why didn't I suspect something when she stopped cooking altogether?) He looked terrible. His stomach was swollen and his face was sallow and sagging. His eyes were lifeless, and he didn't smile, as he always did, when I came in the back door. "Did you go to the flea market today?" I said. He didn't say anything. I looked at her.

"Tell him," she said. For once, she actually looked worried about him.

He still didn't say anything.

"He's been laying around on the floor all week," she said. "And he won't go to the doctor."

"Let's go," I told him. "We're going out to the emergency room." He didn't put up his usual fight. A couple of years earlier, I went down there and he was dragging his right leg around. He said it was "numb." I tried to get him to go to the hospital but he refused. When he didn't like your suggestion, he simply didn't acknowledge it.

Me: "Raymond, why don't you take some of your savings and buy you a lake cottage, so you can fish anytime you want to, without having to worry about having to get a fishing license?"

Raymond: "I heard on the scanner that two old boys had a knife fight out on West Henderson."

The time he had the numb leg, he said he had figured out how to fix that old tractor down at the farm. He got up out of his chair, dragged himself to the door and put on his cap. When I got him inside the truck, I told him he really needed to go to the doctor. "Oh, hell, I probably just had a little old mild stroke," he said. "Would you start the damn truck so we can go?"

He didn't like doctors and hospitals and especially didn't want them to have any of his money. Although he hated the army for the way it treated him and his fellow POWs after the war, he said he would go to the veterans hospital if he had to, rather than let them get their grabbers on any of his money.

But I didn't listen to his protests this time, I took him to the emergency room in Cleburne. When we got to the hospital, he was so weak he could hardly walk. He ignored me when I suggested a wheelchair.

For some reason—Brenda said it was because he didn't have a personal physician—he had to wait for three hours before a staff doctor examined him.

While we were waiting, I said, "If you hadn't smoked, you probably would have lived to be a hundred."

"I know," he said.

After the doctor on call that day finally deigned to examine him, he asked me, "How long has he had kidney problems?" I didn't know.

They catheterized him and admitted him. I called my

mother and told her they were keeping him overnight and to get his things together. I'd be there in a few minutes to pick her up. When I got there, I couldn't understand why she didn't have his things ready. I packed his bag myself but still didn't think it was too unusual. I attributed it to her being upset about his being in the hospital for only the second time in his life.

We stayed till visiting hours were over. He said his feet were cold, so she rubbed them and wrapped them in a blanket. As we were leaving, Raymond gave me his bill-fold. It had about $700 in it. I soon realized why he didn't give it to her. He was all too familiar with the infamous "black hole," as Brenda called it. It was the place where everything disappeared and was impossible to find. Other than being upset about having to stay overnight, he seemed all right when we left. I dropped her off at her house and drove the twenty-five miles home and went to bed. Lindon called the hospital at 11:00 P.M. and the nurse said he was doing fine, that she'd given him a sleeping pill.

At around midnight I got an urgent call to get back to the hospital. He was still alive when we got there, but unconscious. They were doing CPR on him and getting ready to bring in the ventilator. I looked at the monitor. There was no movement. Lloyd, his younger brother, shook his head sadly and said what I was thinking: "When it does that, it means it's all over."

I watched the flurry of hospital personnel for a moment. On their faces was a look of compassionate dis-interest. "Let him go," I said. I was numb with dread but still able to think clearly.

A nurse came up and said, "Do you know what you're saying?"

"He was real tough, with lots of pride," I told her. "He wouldn't want to be hooked up to a machine."

"That's what you want?" she said. "You're sure about that?"

"I want him to get well," I said. "Will that machine do that?"

"No," she said.

So they took the machine away and let him go on out. Congestive heart failure was the official cause of death.

Lindon and Lowell sat with him a while, but I didn't want to. He didn't look like himself. He looked like an old, old man, someone I didn't recognize. His mouth was open and his lips were sucked in and stretched tightly over his toothless gums. Karen and Brenda and I sat with my mother in the family room. She was in shock and just stared dull-eyed at nothing in particular and didn't say anything.

We stayed till morning, then took her home. She fell across the bed on her face, her arms spread out, and cried. "I'll take care of you from now on," I told her.

I've done that, but it almost ruined my health — and my marriage.

CHAPTER NINE

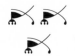

Grandma James lost her mind after Uncle Dock got killed. She threw the medals at the soldiers when they brought them out to the house to give to her. She said she didn't want the insurance money either and called it "blood money." She finally took it, though, and it paid everybody out of debt. Mama drew it for years after Grandma James died. She used to come and stay with us and Daddy was the only one that could do anything with her. Her name was Sarah but he called her Sally. Sometimes she wouldn't come in the house because she said there was a colored man in there. Daddy would go and get an old black coat out of the closet and let her see him taking it out to the shed. "You can come in now, Sally," he'd say. "He's gone for good." Then, she'd come in. She didn't live very long after Uncle Dock died.

At first, during the ten months after Raymond died

that my mother tried to live by herself, it seemed that she was doing it all right. But I didn't realize at the time how often I was making the trip to Cleburne after my classes and on weekends. Brenda and the children began to see the damage it was inflicting on me long before I did.

One of the first things I did was call in the carpenters and give the house a complete makeover — vinyl siding, new carpet, electric stove, new refrigerator, electric water heater, and new wiring. The wiring brought the house up to code. (Though it turned out that the wiring had to be redone later. The local electrician, knowing her condition and that I lived out of town, cheated her.) Every day during the summer when the air conditioner tripped the breaker, Raymond would patiently go around to the back and reset it, probably several times a day. I lack this patience gene. Also, I didn't have the patience, as he did, to relight the pilot on the gas water heater every time someone opened the front door and the air sucked it out. Hence the electric heater. As for the new electric cooking stove, I simply unplugged it and told her it quit working. I did this after she bought a bag of pot-pourri and put it in a pan and set it on fire. "I love the smell of this," she said, "don't you?" as the smoke alarms wailed.

The old porch was torn down and a new, larger one was built, big enough for several people to sit on. I had a hall closet enlarged to accommodate an apartment-sized washer and dryer, the first one she ever had. When it was all finished it was very beautiful but, unfortunately, the work didn't accomplish as much as I thought it would. Her mind couldn't be renovated. She couldn't remember how to use the washer and dryer. She had never learned to use a vacuum cleaner, so that was out. She still unplugged all the appliances and unscrewed all the light bulbs. I had to wash clothes, clean house, cook, and screw the light bulbs back in. She couldn't get to the plug on the refrigerator to unplug it easily, so she just turned the dial down to zero. She couldn't understand why her milk was spoiling. "This milk you buy nowadays," she would say, over and over again, "it just isn't as good as the milk you used to buy. It gets blinky too fast."

Explaining why this was happening was useless, but I did it anyway. Finally, I gave up the lectures, set the dial on medium, and then pulled it off and threw it away.

"I heard the old ladies down the street talking yesterday," she told me one day while the renovation work was going on. "One of them said, 'She must have got a big insurance policy and spent it all on that house.'" This was the first time she ever told me about "the old ladies" who "gossiped" about her. But, of course, I would hear about them ad infinitum in the forthcoming months.

She didn't like anything I had done to the house. The only things she ever praised were the paneling (dark and ugly) that Raymond had nailed up, the curtains, which she picked out, and the wonderful asbestos insulation and plumbing that Raymond had done. "I love my house," she would rhapsodize, "the pretty curtains, the paneling, the insulation, and the good plumbing. That old siding, though, I don't care for. I liked the paint better."

"We could have it torn off. Then you could pay somebody to paint it every year."

"No, I'll just leave it, now that it's already on there."

I told her she needed tires and shocks on her car.

"That car has nearly new tires and shocks. Raymond put them on there just before he died. Don't it set up good? Cars are like old women, they start sagging when they get old. But not this one." (Raymond was too sick to work on cars for the last two years before he died.)

I soon learned all her fetishes. TV clickers, oh, lord, how she used to push me to the edge looking for the TV clicker. The neighbors were coming in the house and stealing them, she told me. Usually I would find it under her pillow or in a drawer. When I refused to look for it anymore, she started buying new ones—at about $25 each. Finally, I epoxyed one to the coffee table. One of the few victories I've had.

Another is keys. She was endlessly losing them, locking herself out of the house or out of her car. One of her neighbors found one set in the street, and he brought another set over one day and said the street sweeper picked them up, after he had run over them. Some of them were bent double.

"Why are my keys bent?" she asked repeatedly.

"The street sweeper ran over them."

"Well, that's not true. How could that happen?"

"You lost them in the street."

"I never lose my keys."

Never mind that the neighbors had to crawl in her window so often they just started leaving an ice pick on the ledge under the carport to use to unlock the window.

Her purse. I played "Find the Purse" so many times that I finally gave up. I took her billfold, containing her driver's license, checks, Medicare card, all her keys, and now keep it with me. "Find the Purse" is devastating to my nerves. It's always the same:

"Where's my purse?"

We look under the mattress.

Not there.

"Well, I don't know what could have happened to it. I

never lose my purse. I always put it in the same place."
Panic. "Oh, my lord. Everything I own in the world is in
that purse. My driving license. My checkbook. I didn't
lose it. Where is it? If you find it, I'll give you a hundred
dollars." Crying. More panic.

In the drawers.

Not there.

In the trunk.

Not there.

In the closets.

Not there.

I give up and go home. The next day, it shows back up.

"Where was it?"

"Where was what?"

"Your purse. You lost it yesterday."

"I never lose my purse."

The black hole again.

Her bills. I had them drafted through her checking
account. When her bank statements come, they include
the bills that have been drafted. They clearly state that
they are not to be paid, as they have been drafted on her
account. She paid them anyway. Several times. The lady
at the cable company said her cable bill was paid up till
the twenty-first century. If present-day bills weren't
enough, she dragged out bills from the 1950s and tried to
pay them.

In addition to ferreting out old bank statements and
other records that Raymond kept, dating back to the
1940s, she is also the curator of records kept by my grandparents, dating to the 1920s. I thought this was all right.
It gave her something to do and kept her out of mischief.
Wrong again. She found an uncashed Medicare check for
$29 made out to my grandmother, who died in 1980, and

took it to the bank and cashed it. I had to go down and make restitution for it when it came back.

Then there was the horror of the insurance check episode.

Someone in the personnel office at Texas Steel called and said Raymond had a $5,000 insurance policy. I took care of all the arrangements and we went up to Fort Worth on May 15, 1992, and picked it up. Then we went to one of her banks in Cleburne and deposited it. Everything went smoothly, I thought, except for a fight we had in the parking lot when she accused me of treating her "like a child" by always doing all the talking in public.

"I try to let you talk," I stammered, "but you never say anything when they ask you questions."

"I do, too!"

"You always look at me. I take that to mean you want me to answer. Then, you always say what I said. It gets on my nerves."

Every day after that, she called me and said there was a check at Fort Worth and we needed to go up there and get it.

At that time, it still wasn't clear to me just how badly off she was. I spent a lot of frustrating hours trying to convince her that we had already done that. "We already got that check. You went with me. We deposited it in the bank."

"There was a woman called me. She said there's a check up there."

Finally, I began to think there really was another check up there. When I called, the lady said, "You already came and picked that up."

Next day. My mother calls and says, "Tommy, a lady called. There's a check up at Fort Worth."

"Nobody called. You dreamed that. I called up there. The lady said she didn't call you. She said we already picked that check up."

"Well, when did we do that? I don't remember it."

"We already did it. It's been deposited."

"Well, I'll just get somebody else to take me."

She started calling Lindon every day. He told her the same thing I told her.

I got a bright idea. I showed her the deposit slip. She took it, and I never saw it again. Black hole.

She got her cousin, Irene Qualls, and her son, Buck, to drive her to Fort Worth. She was going to get the check. She went prepared. She took her marriage license with her. I saw them later. "I hear you took my mother to Fort Worth," I said.

"I'm not sure why," Buck said. "She seemed to think there was a check up there, but they told her she had already picked it up."

"I know," I said.

Later, I told my mother, "I hear that Irene and Buck took you to Fort Worth."

"Buck said I need shocks on my car."

Something like this she can remember.

Although I didn't want her to drive, she did it anyway. Twenty-five miles away, I couldn't do anything to stop her. One afternoon while I was there, she came home looking wild. Her hair was going in all directions. I could tell something happened. "That girl went through the light and nearly hit me," she said.

I went outside and looked at the car. The front fender on the driver's side was bent and there was red paint on her car.

"She did hit you."

"No, she didn't."

"The fender's dented and there's red paint on your car."

"Well, I don't know how it got there."

"Did you get a ticket?"

"No, but that old girl did."

I looked inside her purse. "You didn't get a ticket. You got two tickets. One for pulling out and the other for no insurance. Why didn't you show the officer your insurance card?"

"He didn't ask me for any insurance card."

I looked in her glove box. No card. Black hole again. After that I xeroxed ten copies of her insurance card and placed them in several places in her car, all around the house, and in the freezer.

I called about the citations and was told that if I brought the card in, that particular one would be dismissed. The other one would be, too, if she'd write for her driving record and if it was clear. I did this and told her to be sure to call me when it came in, as it was very important. Otherwise she'd have to pay the ticket and it would make her insurance go up. After four weeks I asked her every day about it. It didn't come, she said.

"Are you sure?"

"I know things like that. It didn't come."

I found the envelope it came in. "Where's the document that came in this envelope?"

"I didn't throw it away."

Black hole.

The court date came and still no driving record. I took her to the city hall and made her write out a check for $65. I was angry because I knew it came in, but I just couldn't find it.

"What are we paying this for?" she said.

"You're paying for that ticket you got."

"What ticket?"

"The one you got when you had that wreck."

"I didn't have any wreck."

"Well, anyway, the policeman says you did and your name is on the ticket. It says you pulled out in front of somebody."

"I'll just have to lay it out in jail. Just take me over to the jail."

"Don't tempt me." (In my mind I said this.)

Months later, I found the driving record. It just appeared, as everything else eventually does, spit out of the black hole.

On January 13, 1993, at about 3:00 P.M., I dropped her off at the garage where the mechanic had put on the new tires and shocks. I called her that night after my classes around 9:00. No answer. I called every thirty minutes until after 11:00. Then I called Raymond's brother, Lloyd, and his wife, Olean. They hadn't seen her. Bobbie and Janey, her neighbors, hadn't seen her. Benny, Janey's husband, went next door and came back and said the lights were all off and the house was locked.

I called the police, and Brenda and I rushed down there. We met the policeman there, and he told us that since she was considered handicapped he could have an APB put out on her. Marty, Bobbie's son, went with me, and we drove up to the cemetery. It was possible that she had driven up there around sundown, had car trouble and didn't know how to get help. Bobbie and her husband, Leo, stayed at the house with Brenda. They said they couldn't go back to bed until we found her. She wasn't at the cemetery, of course. It had been only a desperate guess. When we got back to her house, Lindon, Lowell, and Karen were there. (Karen was especially shaken, as she had ridden the twenty-five miles with Lindon in his 1967 Dodge Charger with one front wheel dangerously close to falling off and rolling into the next county.) We were all afraid the worst had happened. When there is nothing that can be done but wait, the feeling of helplessness is overwhelming.

At around 3:00 A.M. the phone rang. She was in Glen Rose, the officer said, at the Highway Patrol office. Glen Rose is about twenty-five miles west of Cleburne. She was all right, just confused and disoriented.

She was sitting in the office drinking a Coke when we got there. "Well, Tommy, what are you doing here?" she said, with a crooked smile.

"What am I doing here? What are you doing here is the question."

"I'm all right. There's nothing the matter with me. I could have made it back home. Y'all didn't have to drive all the way up here."

"How in the world did you end up in Glen Rose?" I said on the way back. We were in her car.

"Oh, I took a notion I wanted to drive up to Hico and see Raymond's folks up there. I was on my way home. I wasn't lost."

"Raymond's folks up there have been dead for years. Hico? I can't believe this."

"Tommy, don't be mad at me. And don't tell everybody about this. It wasn't anything."

"Wasn't anything? We thought you were dead somewhere. What do you mean, it wasn't anything?"

"I mean don't tell everybody. They'll think I'm crazy."

"How could I keep from telling them? I had to call all of them to see if they'd seen you."

"Don't this car ride good?" she said. "It's been a lot better since Irene's boy told me to get new shocks on it."

Lindon and I stayed till daylight in her house. She popped up out of bed at eight and said, "Well, what are y'all doing here?"

We still don't know exactly why she got lost. Sometimes she said she picked up a friend and gave him a ride over there, then didn't know how to get back. The friend says no. There's no way to know for sure. They are both notorious for preferring fiction over fact.

The messages she left on my machine grew increasingly frantic. Once, she was crying, saying that someone was going to kill her. Brenda and I rushed down there. She had forgotten about leaving the message but later brought the subject up again. Someone left a message on her door that they were going to kill her, she told us. It turned out to be a particularly scary pamphlet with "The Wages of Sin is Death" as its headline, left there by someone selling religion door-to-door.

Because of their concern for the toll all this was taking on me, Karen, Lindon, and Lowell went to her house two weeks later and told her that she was going to have to move to a retirement home. Simply to say she resisted is like saying Crazy Horse resisted at Little Big Horn. She didn't need to move, she said. She was doing just fine the way it was. She was taking care of herself just fine. She did a good deal of yelling and slamming her hand on the table.

"You're not doing it by yourself," Karen told her. "Daddy is taking care of you, washing your clothes, cleaning house, cooking your meals, cutting the grass, taking you to the grocery store, taking care of your bills. He does everything for you. He even calls you every day and reminds you to take your medicine." (This was true, and it was one of the most frustrating of all my duties. At some point, some doctor had told her to take half a blood pressure pill. This had lodged in her brain. When I said it was time to take her Prozac, she would say, without fail, every time, no exception, "I've already taken half a pill." I began to wait for her to say this with horripilating dread. I always hoped that, just once, she wouldn't say it, but she never surprised me.) "It's killing him," Karen went on, "and we can't sit still and let that happen."

Not so, she said. She could take care of herself. She cooks and cleans and drives her car just fine. And that was it as far as she was concerned. "I take my blood pressure medicine," she said. "I take a half a pill."

At midnight, they were still arguing with her. Lowell, the quietest of our children, and the most analytical, had said very little. He got up and started packing her things.

CHAPTER TEN

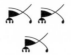

Mama used to tell us about
that boy named Carson Behringer, one of Uncle Dock's friends
when they lived out by Whitney. The one that dove in shallow
water and broke his neck. He like to have died. Uncle Dock
nursed him but he was always paralyzed. Mama said that
"death was furious around his bed." When we were kids
Mama used to tell us all those stories and we would read Uncle
Dock's letters over and over till we almost wore them out.
When she would tell us about Carson Behringer we used to
read his letters to Uncle Dock and look at his picture and feel
sorry for him because he had to sit in that wheelchair. I always
thought he looked awful stiff, like he had a washboard in his
back.

On Sunday, May 30, 1982, Memorial Day weekend,

Lindon dove off a cliff at Waxahachie Lake and broke his neck at the seventh vertebra. The night before, I had driven down to my grandparents' old house in Cleburne to see him. He had moved in after my grandmother died and was still there two months after my grandfather died. It was a drafty old clapboard house with high ceilings and single walls and floors so wavy you almost had to nail the furniture down to keep it from sliding to the other side of the room. My grandparents never cared for insulation. They just heated or cooled one room and closed off the others. The house got so cold at night that the water in the commode froze. I had a turtle once that was quick-frozen in his bowl during one winter night. But no matter how bitter the cold, my grandfather slept out on the back porch, beneath several layers of my grandmother's quilts. "Them old quilts," he said, "and my union suit, is all the insulation I need."

"This old house isn't really fit to live in," I told Lindon. I asked him to move back in with us, and he said he would think about it. We hadn't been getting along very well and he had moved out, first to an apartment, then to my grandparents' house to help my mother see after my grandfather. Lindon said she came over several times every day, cleaning, cooking, trying to make the old man's loneliness bearable.

Lindon told me he had started taking guitar lessons and got up and went into his bedroom and brought out a new guitar and showed it to me. He was tall and muscular and extraordinarily handsome, with a thick black beard. His blue eyes are particularly conspicuous with his long black hair. One of his girlfriends' younger sisters called him "Alabama Man," because he looked so much like the lead singer of the popular singing group Alabama. He showed me a black-powder pistol and holster he had bought the day before at a flea market. He had been practicing his "fast draw," he said.

When I left, he walked me to my truck in the driveway behind his almost-new 1981 Ford pickup. It was a cool evening, and the moon was rising over Mrs. Holt's bungalow on the other side of the garden. You could hear the easy wind shooshing through the giant pecan tree beside the driveway. He told me he'd drop by the next day if Karen didn't set him up with a date. Backing out of the driveway, I stopped and watched him walk away and go back into the house. The old screen door banged shut behind him. For some inexplicable reason, I remember the sorrowful way that old door sounded as it banged shut. Looking back on it, I guess it was closing hard on his past life as we had known it. It would be the last time I would ever see him walk.

The next day his plans to go with Karen and her friends to the lake hadn't worked out and so he called around noon and said he would come by and eat hamburgers with us. He stopped by his former girlfriend's house in Midlothian and talked with her father for a while, then ran into his best friend, Jimmy Wharton, on his way to our house and decided to go out to the lake with him and drink a little beer.

He was four months short of twenty-two and now faced living the rest of his life in a wheelchair. The devastation that careless plunge visited on his life and ours is inexpressible and unimaginable to anyone who hasn't undergone something like it.

For weeks we stayed with him as he lay strapped to a Stryker Frame, unable to move. It was harder to endure than anything I could have ever imagined. At the time, we could see only his great suffering and were given no hope that it would ever get better.

That terrible night, after Karen arrived at the hospital, she and her mother sat on the floor, holding each other and rocking back and forth, like desperate caged animals. Lowell, thirteen at the time, lay on the floor beneath Lindon for hours at a time as he lay on his stomach on the Stryker Frame. At the time this happened, Lowell was a virtuoso trumpet player, winning all the awards in his school contests and an invitation to attend the workshop at Interlochen, in Michigan, a program for gifted young musicians. He didn't attend that or enter another contest. After Lindon's accident, he never played the trumpet again.

Brenda, who had been a registered nurse for ten years, saved Lindon's life on more than one occasion but, most dramatically, one dreadful night when pneumonia clogged him up and the respiratory therapist panicked and couldn't get the tube down. Brenda took over and suctioned him.

This was only one of a series of painful and life-threatening mistakes made by doctors and hospital personnel during his acute stage. The closest they came to killing him was the evening of June 11, 1982. A friend had persuaded me to come over and take a break at his house for a while. Soon after getting there I felt uneasy and rushed back to the hospital with an inexplicable feeling of dread. When I got there, Lindon was unconscious. Two LVNs, each unaware of the other, had injected his forehead with lidocaine. The halo frame, which was bolted into his skull, had been attached improperly, and the pain was so intense he couldn't eat. Before the specialist finally admitted he had screwed the pins in wrong and redid the procedure, they just kept him sedated with painkillers. Luckily, he pulled out of it.

I was the only one he allowed to lift his head and position it on the pillow. The halo frame made it impossible for him to sleep comfortably. It looked like medieval torture equipment. When my mother saw him she held up better than I thought she would. But, outside his room, she cried and said, "Oh, that awful thing, screwed into his pretty head."

She and Raymond stayed at our house most of the time that Lindon was in the ICU, and I took them to see him every day. Raymond said, "I think it might take as long as six months, but I think Lindon will get over this." He and Lindon were fishing buddies and scrap-yard scouts. Lindon always liked to go with Raymond on his forages to the Cleburne Scrap Yard. I couldn't tell Raymond the doctors said it was permanent, but he eventually realized it. My mother never talked about it.

I knew that it was permanent from the first. The night it happened the surgeon told us that the injury was "complete and total." A few minutes later they brought Lindon out of the emergency room on a gurney. When he saw me, he took my hand gently and said, "I messed up, Dad."

There are many misconceptions about spinal cord injuries, the cruelest being that a patient can overcome it if he works hard enough and has "faith," "dedication," and "courage." The spinal cord, enclosed inside the spinal column, is much like the tiny wires inside a telephone cord. If the cord's housing is smashed, a breakdown of transmission can occur, depending on how many wires — or, in the spinal cord, nerves — are damaged. If enough wires remain intact, some communication may still be possible, but there may be lots of static or generally poor reception and transmission. When enough spinal nerves are intact for information to flow between the brain and the rest of the body, the injury is said to be "incomplete," after which the patient recovers in varying degrees. Some, if not all, function will return regardless of what the patient does. The patient could work hard and pray, or lie in the bed and curse God, and it wouldn't matter. Hard work will, of course, rebuild muscles, but only if the nerves are intact. But if the injury is "complete," as in Lindon's case, no amount of determination, prayer, or hard work will have any effect. But, of course, nothing can change this popular misconception. When a patient says, "I'm going to walk out of this hospital" and does it, because the injury is incomplete, only those who have been through it know why.

For a while, I held onto the slim hope that he would recover. I read everything on the subject. I talked to doctors and researchers all over the country, trying to find out about all the latest experimental drugs and techniques. I even talked to quacks. One told me he had developed a remedy that worked, something that you drank. He was willing to bargain with me on the cost. That's when I came to my senses and hung up. But I wasn't willing to admit the finality of it. I went into a rage when I heard that one of the seemingly endless number of doctors who came out of nowhere to cash in on his two medical policies told him he would never walk again.

It was Thomas Townson, Lindon's boyhood friend, who first prepared me for the probability that Lindon would always be handicapped. He was also the first to use that word. Maybe it was because Thomas was blind that I accepted it from him without an argument.

When Thomas came in from Austin to visit Lindon in

the hospital I took him into the room and led him to the Stryker Frame where Lindon lay upside down. "What's going on?" Thomas said, his usual greeting. He is slender, wide-shouldered, and a shock of tan hair spills over his forehead.

"I broke my neck, Tommy," Lindon said. "They've got me strapped in."

"Where is the boy?" Thomas said, turning toward me. I had forgotten to tell him Lindon was upside down. The nurse came and switched him right-side-up, and Thomas moved his fingers along the bolts and pins of the halo frame. His jaw quivered and he winced as he placed the tips of his fingers on the sites where the pins were screwed into Lindon's forehead. He felt of Lindon's feet and pinched his toes. "Can you feel that?" he said.

"Tommy, you could chop off my legs with an axe and I wouldn't feel it," Lindon said.

The two of them had been inseparable during their school years, even in college, where they were room-mates. Lindon helped Tommy with his books and read his lessons to him. They were also known around campus for their occasional fights. "I could hold my own with him," Lindon said, "as long as I could keep him from getting his hands on me. Nobody could whip him at wrestling."

Lindon took him everywhere with him after he got a car. Thomas bought a flat-bed truck and they went into the hay-hauling business. After Thomas went off to the State School for the Blind at Austin, Lindon drove down and picked him up for the weekend or met him at the bus station. Later, when Thomas moved to Houston and went into the concessions business at NASA, Lindon met him at the airport on weekends and brought him home.

After his accident, Lindon still drove down and picked

Tommy up on weekends or met his plane at the airport. They drew stares as Tommy held onto Lindon's wheelchair and followed him through the airport, but it didn't bother Lindon. "Why not?" he said. "It is a pretty weird sight, you have to admit." In their thirties now, they're still friends, though they still have their battles. Of all his friends, Lindon says he's most comfortable with Tommy because he can't see him the way he is now in contrast with the way he used to look.

After Lindon was released from the hospital, I tried to protect my mother as much as I could from the terrible realities of his day-to-day care. Several times, I had come home from class and found him on the floor, wedged between the commode and the wall, or on the driveway, where he had fallen after trying to get into his truck. But one day, I came home and found her and Raymond sitting in the kitchen. She was crying. I went into his bedroom and found him lying in a twisted knot, clinging to the only dry spot on the bed. His catheter had come loose and he was unable to reinsert it. He told them to stay outside his room, that I would be home soon and would take care of it.

Which I did. Afterwards, I reached down to hug him and started crying. "I can't stand it that you're hurt so bad," I sobbed.

"Well, that's just the way it is," he said.

I felt terrible, doing this to him, breaking down and having to be comforted by a boy who had been physically and mentally wrecked.

I am writing this chapter on Memorial Day. As he always does, Lindon called today and said he had just come in from the lake—with Jimmy, of course. Jimmy's brother had bought a new jet ski and Lindon had taken it for a few turns around the lake (not at breakneck speed, he said). He was also quick to say that he wore a life jacket—"I didn't want to drown on Memorial Day." He told me he feels fortunate—that he didn't die, that he has family and friends, that he has his own home and didn't have to go to a nursing home. It took over twelve years before he was able to say that.

My mother's usual way of dealing with problems by denying them didn't work with Lindon's accident—denial was impossible. It was the third undeniable blow she had suffered in two years. On December 1, 1980, my grandmother had died suddenly of a heart attack. My grandfather died sixteen months later. He had a heart problem, too. It was broken.

The loss of her parents was the greatest tragedy of my mother's life. Brenda thinks her attachment to them was so obsessive that she was never able to end her grief and resume her life. Chronic depression, she says, can cause dementia. Then Lindon's accident came. Soon after that, she had to face the death of Brad Johnson, the eighteen-year-old son of neighbors Benny Earl and Janey. She and Raymond were distraught to lose the boy they had baby-sat since he was born. She spent much more time with him than she ever had with me.

There is no way now to know how much misery she must have put Raymond through in the years since the early 1980s. After only two years of caring for her, I was in the hospital twice. During that time I had diarrhea every day. In August of 1993 I was having lunch with Brenda and Lowell when I suddenly started having chills. I went outside to warm up. It was a hundred degrees outside, but I was still shivering. That evening my temperature went up to 104. I was in bed, and Brenda was watching television in the other end of the house. I wanted to get up out of bed but couldn't will myself to do it. I lay there, hoping the telephone would ring and it would be for me, so she would come and see that I was on my way to that great classroom in the sky. I couldn't even call out loudly enough for her to hear me. Finally, she came to bed. She took a look at me, took my temperature and went into emergency mode. Tylenol brought my temperature down, but the next day I was in the hospital for tests. One was an intestinal photo opportunity in which I was fundamentally skewered by an optical apparatus I called the Amazing Butt Weasel. For an x-ray session I was pumped full of Portland cement, though the nurse insisted on calling it barium. Because I survived these treatments, the doctors apparently decided that nothing could kill me and sent me home. Their diagnosis was that I had diverticulitis resulting from "stress." My doctor told me, "We used to call it 'nervous stomach.'"

My mother told everybody I had the "piles."

"It's not the piles! It's stomach trouble!"

"Daddy used to say he got the piles from riding the harrow."

"It's not the piles. It's a stomach disorder caused by stress."

"I didn't know you had that. How come you have that?"

"I don't want to talk about it."

I ran into Raymond's brother, Lloyd, after that and he said, "How's your piles?"

When she couldn't get hold of me on the phone to tell me her troubles she called Lindon and told him. She usually said she wanted to die. I was furious when I found this out. He lived day to day with the severest of problems. He has chronic unrelenting pain in one of his arms and in his side. He has chronic urinary tract infection. It takes him over an hour just to get out of bed each day and get dressed. Every other week he has to change his catheter tube, which goes through his groin directly into his bladder, a painful procedure requiring heavy painkillers just to get it done.

Of course, it was because of her dysfunction that she did this, but I wasn't able at that time to make those allowances. Sometimes, as with the condom incident, I still can't. I told her not to call him and do this to him. "Poor Lindon," she would say, with the sincerest of conviction. "Bless his heart, I know he suffers so." And then do the same thing again the next day.

He was the one who had the most time to help me with her. Karen teaches full-time, and Lowell, a field engineer, works twelve-hour shifts. Karen also has Haylee and Beth to care for. So, Lindon took my mother to the doctor when I couldn't do it, or to get groceries, or to the cemetery. Once, he took her to a Stamps Quartet concert, which she greatly enjoyed but had no recollection of by the time they got to the car. It's awfully hard to ask him, or the other children, to do things like this for her when you know she won't remember them.

Sometimes I can't help comparing my role as "caregiver," to use the current lingo, with Lindon and now with her. Caring for Lindon when he was in the acute stage was exhausting mentally, emotionally, and physically, but it wasn't as hard as this has been. At the time I didn't think anything could be as bad. During the year he lived with us before he got his own place, Brenda and I helped him with his every need, even his toilet needs. We had to help him transfer in and out of his wheelchair. We catheterized him. We helped him put on his shoes and stockings, change clothes, bathe. I was a sounding board for his rage. But, despite all this horror and pain and knowledge that he was never going to get back to the way he was, it was endurable because at least he was going to live, and also because he appreciated it and told us so in a thousand ways, with words and sometimes just with a look. He still does. Though he has improved to the point where he doesn't need much help, simple things like cutting the grass or even changing the sheets on his waterbed are impossible for him. When I help him install spark plugs or a water pump or do any other chore that used to be easy for him, I know there's no question that he would be doing the same for me if the situation were reversed. There's never been any doubt about that in my mind.

With her, it's much harder. Alzheimer's victims are generally unable to understand a kindness. After I cut her grass, she usually says, "A boy came and mowed my lawn." When I had the new tires and shock absorbers put on her car, she said, "Raymond put those on there before he died." And so on. Sometimes I didn't have the strength for it and avoided seeing her or talking to her for a week at a time.

After Raymond died, I had her bills drafted on her account and my name placed on the accounts to prevent thieves (such as the dishonest Cleburne electrician) from conning her out of her money. She can't write a check or withdraw money without my signature. She can't keep up with her checkbook and usually hands it to the salesperson to make out the check. Most of the time, she lays it down in the store and walks away. She often accuses me of taking her money. And her house. And her purse. And her keys. And her TV clicker.

Even her marriage license. "Where's my marriage license?" she says, totally out of the context of anything imaginable.

"I don't know."

"You had it."

"I didn't ever have it. What would I want with your marriage license?"

It was no use. I had taken it from her and I couldn't convince her otherwise.

Finally, I hunted it down and found it in a drawer. I took it and had ten copies made and put them in her purse, in her drawer, in her car, and in the refrigerator. I felt immensely vindicated.

"I never said you got it," she said.

It isn't natural being the parent of your mother. I felt guilty for taking over her finances but, if I hadn't, some-one probably would have stolen everything from her by now. I wonder about the demented homeless elderly. How many of them had money and a home at one time and lost everything to con artists or even thieving family members and ended up on the street? When I tell her that I've heard of children doing this to their parents, she says she's sorry and that she does appreciate me and everything I've done for her. Then, next day, same thing. She even told a neighbor once, "I wish I had a daughter so I'd have some-body to take care of me."

CHAPTER
ELEVEN

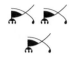

W e moved around a lot
when Daddy was farming. After we left Egan we moved to the
Long place between Joshua and Cleburne. The Hudsons lived
not too far from us. Their house was falling down and made
ours look pretty good. We were farming on the halves then and
they were farming on the fourths. They were nice though.
They had a daughter named Janetta. Then we moved out to
the Carruthers place between Joshua and Godley. Steve and
Aunt Bessie lived down the road from us. Bessie and Aunt
Annie married brothers, Steve and Adell. Their kids were double cousins. Annie was quiet, like Daddy. And she suffered
with the sugar diabetes. But Bessie was always stubborn and
her and Steve used to fight like cats and dogs. She used to tell
everybody she was going out on dates with Gene Autry. She'd

come to our house and say, "Well, Gene called and said he
wanted me to meet him in Fort Worth at the Fat Stock Show
but it makes Steve so mad when I do, that it just ain't worth
it." After she'd leave, Daddy would say, "Gene Autry
wouldn't look at her. She knows better than that." Those were
good old days, though. I didn't mind all the moving around
because I always wanted to see what kind of house we were
going to have next. And no matter how far we got out in the
sticks, Mama always found a church and a school for us to go
to. I didn't go but to the seventh grade but I won the prize for
best penmanship.

Two weeks after she got lost in Glen Rose, we loaded
her up and moved her, over her angry objections, to the
retirement home. Brenda was horrified when she took the
sheets off her bed. They were black with grime. Brenda
said they probably hadn't been changed in five years or
more. There were seventeen unopened bottles of cooking
oil in her pantry and fourteen pounds of margarine in her
refrigerator. She had fifteen full boxes of aluminum foil.
Now, when I take her to the grocery store, she moves
toward these items as though drawn by a magnet. She
reaches for the cooking oil.

"Don't even think about it," I say.

The retirement home is an attractive building in the
center of a huge parcel of well-kept acreage. The large
reception room where the residents — mainly women, but
a few couples and an occasional single man — congregate
before meals and in the evening to gossip has a grand
piano, several large chandeliers, and a spiral staircase.
There is a dining room with elegant furnishings and fine
dishes and tableware. Her upstairs apartment had a back

view overlooking a meadow where goats and horses graze. Reluctantly, she watched as we moved her in on that rainy January 29, 1993.

We were apprehensive, so I stayed in her apartment with her the first night, hoping to soften the shock of waking up the next morning and finding herself in strange surroundings.

It didn't help. The next morning she said, "I have a couch just like that."

"It is your couch," I said.

"What's my couch doing here?" she asked me. "And I've got a picture just like that one." She pointed to an oil painting of the farmhouse Raymond was born in.

"Yours, too," I said. "This is all your furniture. We moved you in here yesterday."

"I've got to go home."

She stayed, but for six months she begged me every night on the phone to go home. "These old ladies," she would say, "they pretend to be so good, but they're really not. They talk about me behind my back." Lots of tears. "I pray every night that you'll let me go back home."

"Which ones?" I would say. "Which ones are doing these things? I see you talking to them every evening that I visit you. You seem to be enjoying it, you're laughing and talking. You love the meals. Who's doing these things to you?"

She couldn't say. Just the "old ladies." Actually, the residents were all friendly and receptive to her and helped her in every way possible to adjust. Other than an occasional complaint by the director that "Juanita loses her keys seventeen times a day," the administrators seemed to think she was doing fine. There were activities, gossip, outings, and games. On Thursdays they went to the beauty college and to Wal-Mart in the van. But it just couldn't work. Those "old ladies."

To pacify her, I left her car parked under the far end of the pavilion so that she could see it from her window. The director told me that my mother went out and started it up every day. This was her favorite occupation, other than begging to go home.

Unfortunately, her unconcern for news events didn't apply to the government's war against the Branch Davidians at Mount Carmel. As the victims were oblique Seventh-Day Adventists, the church which owns and operates the retirement home, she and her contemporaries watched every terrible episode of that senseless tragedy on television. They were watching as the compound exploded and incinerated everyone inside, including seventeen children. After this, she seemed more agitated and fearful than ever before. In her paranoid state, she may have been afraid that tanks were going to come and push down her walls and set her building on fire. I asked her about that and she said she wasn't afraid. But I didn't quite believe her. I think she minimizes her real fears as she hyperbolizes her imagined ones. I tried to assure her that this wouldn't happen, that the government wouldn't attack the retirement home unless the "old ladies" started stockpiling AK-47s.

The regularity of the life there was good for her. She needed the scheduled meals, the organized activities, the socialization. Her childhood ability to play dominoes surfaced. I never saw her play, so I couldn't say whether she was really playing or just throwing the dominoes around. But, at the same time she seemed to be improving, actually enjoying her new surroundings, she was calling me every night, complaining about the "old ladies" who were "gossiping" about her and coming into her room and taking her clicker. Sometimes, she overheard "two old men" talking about her as she walked down the hall. They always commented on her "nice figure." They said, "Why is she in here? She's too young to be in a place like this."

I always thought "paranoia" was simply an institutional term used to label and control citizens with an acute sense of consciousness, in other words, suspicious and cautious people. I believed that when such people became nuisances to their family or to the state, they were diagnosed, overmedicated and, sometimes, institutionalized. Paranoia, I believed, was simply a useful term designed to control smart people. I had observed that this label was often leveled at artists, philosophers, leaders of social movements, and the like. These people, I reasoned, are naturally going to be cautious and suspicious of other people, institutions, even the government. But paranoia, I now believe, is more than a heightened sense of self-consciousness. It is the result of a brain dysfunction that can strike anyone, from Ernest Hemingway to my mother, who probably never had an artistic or political theory in her life. When we find ourselves the target of such irrational fears or the caregiver of someone so afflicted, we should perhaps find strength in the old adage, "Here but for the grace of God go I" and, if possible, remember mercy.

CHAPTER
TWELVE

When we were little, Grandma James would go around and stay with all her kids. She would come and stay for several weeks at a time with us. It was funny. She wouldn't but just get there when she would say she had to go. She'd go out to the barn and get up in the buggy and say she had to go to George's place—that was Uncle Jack. Nobody could do anything with her except Daddy. He'd go out to the barn and say, "Now, Sally, I'll take you down to Jack's in the morning. Now, you get out of that buggy and come on in the house and go to bed." She'd get out of the buggy and do what he said. Next morning, she'd forgot all about wanting to go to Uncle Jack's till it started getting dark. Then, she'd start it up again about needing to go. I guess Daddy had to do that every night.

The six months my mother spent at the retirement

home were the easiest time for me since Raymond died. I didn't have to go take care of her every day and could visit when I wanted to. Sometimes I'd pick her up and take her to the cemetery, driving through Egan on the way. Egan was always her cue for a long stroll down memory lane. But she enjoyed those trips—and so did I. Her new home was five miles closer to our house, so one of us would drive down and get her and bring her to our house on special occasions. Unfortunately, though, she was always ready to go back as soon as she got there. "Well, Tommy, I guess I'd better be going back," she'd say, even before she sat down. "The old ladies lock the door at sundown."

I enjoyed that entire six months. I actually had some time to myself and could think about something other than her and her problems. The dream about the key in the trunk faded from my subconscious for the entire period.

One of her problems—actually my problem—was a friend she talked to on the telephone every evening. They had been doing this for over forty years, since they worked together at Duke & Ayres in Cleburne. Understandably, her friend didn't want her to move, but her reaction was over the edge. She began a campaign calculated to undermine our plans, and she wouldn't be satisfied until my mother returned to her house in Cleburne. She became an incubus. She apparently told my mother that I just wanted her in that place so that I could take over her house and finances and keep her from driving. The incubus even told me once on the telephone that my mother didn't need to be in that "nursing home," that there was nothing wrong with her. I asked her if she would like to drive to Glen Rose at four in the morning to retrieve her the next time she got lost. "If you'll be responsible for her, clean and cook, cut her grass, and screw all the light bulbs back in every day, I'll be glad to let her move back," I said. She said she couldn't do that, that her health was bad, that she had been having this awful pain in her feet, blah blah blah.

Bobbie, the neighbor across the street, said that the incubus drove by every day to check on my mother's house. One day when Brenda and I dropped by my mother's apartment, she had obviously been talking to the incubus on the phone. I could tell she was agitated. Suddenly, she said, "Who's living in my house!" "Nobody," I said. Since this was before I learned of the "Good Old Days" technique, we drove her back there to prove to her that no one was living in her house. By the time we got there, she had forgotten she ever said it.

At first, we didn't understand why she had gotten such a thing into her head, then we remembered that we had stopped by there earlier to check on things, and the incubus had driven by and seen my wife's car, which she suspected was owned by the "new tenants."

The incubus told Bobbie that her children tried to put her in a nursing home, but she wouldn't go. She has never had any children. Bobbie said she started hanging up on the incubus when she called.

Finally, the pleading broke me down and I gave in. She could go home if she would promise to sign up for Meals on Wheels and weekly housekeeping. "Oh, yes, yes, yes!" she said, "Oh, thank you thank you thank you. My prayers have been answered."

The move was too much for me this time, so I hired two boys to do it. My mother was ecstatic. She would soon realize, however, that just because she moved back to her house, she wasn't going to have it the way it was before Raymond died.

She wanted to start driving again. No, Brenda advised me. It was too dangerous. Her driver's license had expired, and I hoped she wouldn't want to renew it—no such luck. The incubus called and reminded her that she needed to get that done. Don't take her to get it renewed, Brenda said. If you do, she said, at least tell them she needs to take another test. But I gave in and took her. My mother was enraged about this driver's license business and yelled at me all the way to the Department of Public Safety. As soon as we walked inside, however, her attitude changed from rage to charm. Her photo on the license looks like someone who has just won the lottery.

I didn't tell them they had just renewed the license of an Alzheimer's patient. No one asked, and I kept my mouth shut. I reached deep inside my rationality file. What came up was: "I'm not renewing her license. The state is. So the state is responsible for her." I went down that afternoon and increased her auto liability to the maximum limit.

She soon lost the weight she had gained at the retirement home, and the delusions got worse. At the grocery store, she whispered, "See that old man? That's old man Doty. I heard him talking to himself after we walked by. He didn't know I could hear him. He said, 'It sure didn't take her long after Raymond died to get another man,'" meaning me, of course. The oedipal implications of this delusion gave me the horripilating fantods. She repeated this story so many times that I finally told her I didn't want to hear it anymore, that it upset me. She also said somebody came in the house and took a jar of pennies she used as a doorstop. "I saw the boy next door looking at it one day," she said. I found the jar of pennies hidden in her closet.

She fixated on the ceiling fan in the living room. It wasn't hers, she said. Somebody, meaning me, had taken her pretty one and left this ugly one. "This is the one that has always been in this house," I told her. "You're thinking about the one you had at your apartment."

"No," she explained, her blue eyes blazing. "This is not mine. Now where is mine? I want to know! You tell me!"

"No one can tell you anything." I said this in my mind, of course. What I really said was, "Okay, let's go out to Wal-Mart and buy another one." I picked out one like the one she remembered from her apartment and left it in her kitchen, still in the box, until Lowell could come down and help me install it.

That evening, she called and said she was scared. There was a fan on her porch, in a box, and she didn't know where it came from. Somebody had put it there to scare her.

"It's the one we bought at Wal-Mart."

"Oh, no, I didn't buy that. Somebody put it there to scare me. Now, why would anybody do that? I'm going to call the police."

I figured she had put the offending fan on the porch and forgot she did it. She throws out everything she thinks isn't hers. "No," I said, "don't call the cops. I'll come down and get rid of it." I returned it and got her money back.

She didn't change her clothes for days at a time. I instructed the housekeepers to wash her clothes, but I couldn't be there in the mornings to make sure she put on clean clothes. I had a hairdresser come to her house and take care of her hair when I realized that she wasn't washing it. I had extra keys made and placed them in several locations around the house. I took her grocery shopping every Friday. I thought everything was working out. But I didn't realize that I was falling back into my old pattern of going down there several times a week. Brenda felt neglected and became increasingly angry and resentful.

After my mother had been back at home for about six months, the police began calling me. They said she called them several times a day. "Somebody came in my house and stole my purse," she told them. In other words, every time she forgot where she hid it. An officer would have to come out and help her play "Find the Purse." I promised I would do something about this. Of course, she denied she ever did such a thing. "I have never lost my purse!" she said indignantly.

After that, she started calling 911. She did this several times a day. Once, she called 911 and said something was wrong with her phone. The worst thing she did, the thing that almost got me in a rage, was when she called the cops and told them that I came and took her car keys and "gouged out the ignition" so she couldn't drive her car.

I rushed down there, as usual. I didn't bring it up about the cops. She was already agitated enough. I just asked her why she thought I gouged out her ignition. "I didn't say you gouged it out," she said. "I said somebody gouged it out."

"The ignition is worn out! The car's fifteen years old, for God's sake! Things wear out!"

"Oh, no, it's not worn out. Raymond kept that car in perfect condition."

I had a wrecker come and haul it to the Ford dealership. "Ignition's worn out," the mechanic said.

"Would you tell this to my mother?" I said.

"Ignition's worn out," he said.

"I never said it wasn't," my mother said calmly.

"I know," I said. "You said I gouged it out."

That's when she went into her nervous overload mode. When she does this, it's scary. She turns her body sideways to you, doubles up her fists and affects a kind of blustering posture; old-timers called it "bowing up" to you (that's "bow" as in bow and arrow). Then she says something like, "Oh, lord, I wish I could die. I think I'll take strychnine." Her face contorts and her voice gets garbled, like the little girl's in *The Exorcist*.

The final straw this time (where is that camel of last resort that bears all the final straws?) was when the police called one afternoon, just after I had gotten home from a particularly stressful day at work. "What did I do now?" I said.

"You broke into her house."

"Then what?" I asked.

"You took everything she had in her old trunk."

I would have pulled all my hair out if it hadn't fallen out already.

I could feel myself breaking down. But I somehow thought a trip to the doctor would help her. I couldn't take her—at this point I didn't want to ever see her again. Lindon volunteered to take her. Besides, I had taken her so many times before, to so many different doctors, hoping for some miracle. It was always the same:

"Who's the president, Juanita?"

"Uh, Carter?"

"What year is it?"

"Nineteen eighty-two?"

"How old are you?"

"Let me see ... sixty-four? I was born in 1918."

The session always ends with the doctor telling me to watch her bathroom habits, get her an I.D. bracelet, and label everything in the house — all textbook stuff. Sometimes the doctors changed her medication. Once, for six weeks, I got her on the "Cognex" program when it was still experimental. Forty percent of those taking it had improved dramatically, I was told. Others were helped in lesser proportions, and some not at all. I paid Lloyd and Olean's daughter, Elaine, $50 a week to drive over to her house and give it to her four times a day. I arranged for a home-health nurse to come weekly and test her for liver damage, a possible side effect of the drug. There was no change that I could see and discontinued it.

On this particular visit, Lindon said that when the doctor asked her why she was calling the police so much she drew back her hand and the doctor thought she was going to deck him. But she was just raising her hand to swear that this was a foul and odious lie, that she had never called the police in her life.

Later, when I found the strength, I talked to her about this police thing. I didn't want to tell her never to call 911, as there might be a real emergency some day. But I wanted her to stop calling them about her "missing" purse and other imagined felonies. She said she had never done such a thing, but if she had she would never do it again. "I promise," she said.

The following evening, after I had just gotten home from my night classes, tired and just wanting to watch a little TV and go to bed, the phone rang. It was Janey Johnson, her neighbor next door. "Tommy, Nita's hurting real bad with her back. She's on the couch and can't get up. I didn't know what to do so I called you."

Oh lord, I thought.

"Okay," I told her. "Thanks for calling. I'll come down and check on her."

When I got there she was still on the couch, and Janey was seeing after her. "I'm going to take you to the emergency room," I told her. "You'll get a shot and it will relieve you."

"Oh, I'll be all right in a few days," she said. "It's just this old sciatical nerve. I've had it before. Mama had it. I guess I inherited it from her."

I don't think she expected this emergency room idea, but she got up and hopped dramatically to the car. I drove her thirty-five miles to Baylor Hospital at Waxahachie. Brenda is the director of the ICU there and could make everything smooth for us.

During the forty-minute drive, she didn't mention her back except to say that it "feels a lot better."

Oh lord.

Brenda stayed on after her shift to meet us there. She helped my mother into the waiting room and helped her complete her medical forms. She stayed with her in the emergency room and introduced her to the doctor. He gave her a shot and some pills and she was fine. On the way back home, she said, "Is Brenda working? I never see her anymore."

It was after midnight by the time I got to bed. This was the last time I would ever drive to Cleburne to see after her, I vowed. And it was, but it wouldn't be the last time I would have to contend with the dread "sciatical nerve."

Soon after that is when I noticed that the house across the street was available.

CHAPTER THIRTEEN

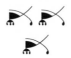

Ⅰf anybody should never been sent to the war, it was Uncle Dock, Mama said. He wasn't like the other boys. Family was everything to him. He'd rather stay at home and talk to the girls than go around to dance halls and things like that. He had a girlfriend, though, named Ethyl Biffle, from Meridian, that he took to church. She wrote to him after he went to the war. We have some of her letters to him and a picture of her in that old trunk. The government sent it all to us after he was killed. We never knew exactly what happened but we heard that a shell exploded and killed him and the horse he was riding.

Does a fatherless boy spend his life looking for heroes?

If so, this may explain my childhood need to attach myself to older boys and, later, to "father figures." Bill Leonard, an older boy from the neighborhood, now a lawyer in Cleburne, must have wondered what mortal sin he had committed to have a molecule like me attaching itself to him. There I was, every morning, waiting for him to unlock his father's Studebaker so that I could squeeze myself inside for a ride to school no matter how many of his own friends he had to carry. He protected me more than once, however, from the beatings I used to receive with regularity from Darrell Walker, another older boy from the neighborhood and an unlikely prospect for a hero by anybody's definition other than my own.

Later, I discovered the idlers who hung out at the Cleburne Shoe Shop, former high school football stars whose luster had paled considerably over the years. Because I was ten years younger than the youngest of these Runyonesque characters, I was never acknowledged by any of them as a living entity and occupying space, much less accepted as a member of their exalted order, no matter how much I longed for it. It was a closed society. It began in Cleburne High School in the 1940s and wasn't accepting any new members. Among them, working for wages seemed to be a stumbling block for ascension into leadership positions within the hierarchy. The few with steady jobs were railroaders. The others were day laborers and gamblers. They had names like "Hod," "Biggy," "Skyblue," "Abie," and "Coot."

The one I revered most was Ralph Junell, the fearsome "leader" of the "shoe-shop gang." It was indicative of his status that he was the only one without a nickname. Nicknames imply vulnerability, intimacy and, sometimes, endearment — attributes no one would ever associate with him. His round, pleasant appearance masked a rough and cynical indifference rooted, it was said, in the disappointment of a long-ago football injury that derailed his train to college gridiron fame. His loose-fitting lightweight slacks, loafers, and sport shirts, always open at the collar and outside his pants, denoted a fashion statement: "I'm smooth, silent, and lethal."

Women who came into the shop with their shoes in their hands forgot why they came in if he was in there. They would forget their change or even to pick up their repaired shoes. Sometimes they gave him diamond rings or other precious tokens of their love. Other than "jeweler," his main occupation was gambling. The only real job he apparently ever had was in the late 1950s, when he was said to be the bodyguard for the widow of Edele Evans, the Fort Worth mobster found stuffed in a well near Godley.

A hello from this swarthy, sullen small-town boulevardier would have sent me into paroxysms of joyous howling dithyrambs. I would have settled for an insult. But a consistent silent disdain was wounding beyond all injuries. I told myself his hard exterior covered a soft heart. I had read too many Steinbeck novels.

As his reflexes slowed, a lot of young bar brawlers were watching. Eventually, he was badly beaten up and his leg broken by a heavyweight champion Golden Gloves boxer, it was said, in a bar fight at Fran's Cove on Berry Street in Fort Worth.

Ramon "Doc" McDearmon, the proprietor of the Cleburne Shoe Shop, was also the unofficial advocate for this cadre of wayward boys, myself included. These "charter members" came because Doc was one of the town's biggest Yellow Jackets supporters and had decorated his walls with pictures of them in uniform. Most of them were rounded up by the draft board officer and sent to Korea in 1950. Doc said the shop was a lonely place for a couple of years.

They met there every morning, read the sports pages, and planned the day's activities. If there was no card game somewhere, they usually spent summer afternoons listening to the baseball game before loading into someone's car for an evening at Berry Street's Twilight Lounge or the Jungle Lounge, later Fran's Cove. Doc, a deacon in the Church of Christ, never drank or gambled. He did, however, smoke several packs of Phillip Morris a day and drink coffee all day long from a pint milk bottle. His face was crisscrossed with cigarette furrows and accented by a medium-sized strawberry nose. His hands were permanently stained with forty years of shoe dye and nicotine. I saw him only a couple of times without his apron, and when I did, I thought he didn't look like himself. I used to sit and watch him peel, scrape, carve, hammer, sew, glue, and buff new life into old shoes.

Sometimes when a customer brought in a pair of shoes, Doc would look at them briefly and say, "Not worth fixing. Buy a new pair."

"Doc, you know she'll just take them down the street to the other guy's shop and get them fixed," I said. "You might as well fix them yourself."

"Gotta sleep at night," was all he said.

He gave me a totally different way of looking at the world from what I had learned from my mother. For her, appearances were everything. I told him that she didn't like me hanging around his shop and that she didn't exactly approve of his friends. He said, "These boys might knock your teeth down your throat if you crossed them, but they won't stab you in the back. A lot of church members and respected business leaders will do that, though. The boys don't care much for the official law, but they usually shoot pretty straight with each other. I've been letting them slide with a few dollars here and there since they were kids and they always pay me back. I've got customers, church members—they pick up their shoes and say they forgot their billfold and I never see them again. It's just all in the way you look at it."

Doc had a heart attack and died in the mid-1970s, behind his counter, resoling someone's shoes. Most of the old gang showed up for his funeral. I saw Ralph and spoke to him. As always, he ignored me. He died soon after that, too. I would have gone to his funeral if I had known about it.

Then, there was the mayor, another great hero and sponsor of an entirely different "gang," one in which I was welcome. Walter Holliday was generally considered one of the best mayors Cleburne ever had, an honest businessman who had made and given away several fortunes and, more important, a hero to every Cleburne boy who knew him, as well as to his own children, Lonnie and Carol. They brought their high school friends home after school and it became their second home. I was lucky enough to have been one of them. The mayor was a tall and gentle bear-like man with a soft whispery voice and bushy eyebrows. He wore his trousers high, above his girth, in the manner of well-dressed men of that era. He made everyone feel comfortable, welcome, and equal. Rich or poor, star athlete, bench-warmer or nonathlete, valedictorian or class dunce, all were treated with respect. Good things to eat and drink were always around, and the mayor and Mrs. Holliday usually gathered around the dining room table with us for a game of gin rummy, hearts, or poker. On weekends the games usually lasted all night. "Last one out turn out the lights," the mayor would say, on his way upstairs to bed. Typically, my mother never seemed to know of my membership in this club. If she did, she never mentioned it.

In 1988 I received an invitation to return to the Hollidays' one last time for an evening of cards and visiting with the old gang because the Hollidays were moving to a new house. About thirty of us showed up; some of us hadn't seen each other since the old days. We had become lawyers, doctors, railroaders, teachers, realtors, businessmen, dentists. Everyone had, in my opinion, made good.

At the reunion, there was no formality, no agenda, and no one made a speech. Except for some receding hairlines and extended waistlines, everybody seemed the same as ever. The ones who won all the money in the old days won again; the same losers lost, and the kibitzers of old were—you guessed it—still looking over our shoulders and giving unwanted advice. Old complaints re-surfaced. A former halfback was heard to say to a lineman of yore, "You never deal me any good cards—and you wouldn't block for me either!"

It wasn't until his funeral in 1993 that most of us learned the extent of the mayor's generosity. One of the mayor's original protégés, Joe Stephens, gave the eulogy. He told this story: the pastor of the Methodist church had asked the mayor if the church could buy his house and surrounding property. "No," the mayor told him. "I won't sell it to you for any price."

The preacher's disappointment showed in his face.

"I said I wouldn't sell it to you," the mayor said. "But, of course, I'll be happy to give it to you."

We also learned that he had donated other properties to several churches—all of different denominations. What he gave us boys was a sense of egalitarianism, charity, and fair play. Like Doc, he left the moral judgments to the hypocrites.

My first hero, of course, was Andrew Jackson James, my mother's Uncle Dock, written up in the *Fort Worth Star-Telegram* in 1918 as "the first Johnson County boy killed in the Great War." Though he died twenty-one years before I was born, I knew I wanted to be like him because everybody spoke of him with great love and respect. He was my grandmother's twin brother. She never stopped telling my mother and me about him.

In his photographs he looks eerily like Woodrow Wilson, the president Grandma James blamed for his death.

There are thirty-five letters archived in "that old trunk," brown and fragile, written on YMCA or Red Cross stationery chronicling the final six months of his life. He continually urged his mother not to worry, that he would be home someday. To my grandmother, he wrote comforting words, assuring her that she would someday understand the reason for little Howard's death ("I'll never forget how he was burning up with fever when I placed that last kiss on his cheeks," he wrote), that my grandfather's health would improve, and that they would get out of debt. He wondered about his new colt: "Is it large enough to ride? I would give anything in the world to see it." In one letter, he asked for a picture of it.

For his father, he described all the farms he saw from the window of his troop train, the tobacco crops of North Carolina and the large tomato fields in New Jersey: "They would make your eyes bug out of your head." He described the big cities: "I have seen New York, the largest city in the United States. I have seen one steamboat. I have crossed a river of about four miles, I guess." He was puzzled by the zoos: "They have big parks up here," he wrote, "that are full of nothing but animals."

Each letter described a new wonderment, but they all had one common theme: he had great hope that he would come back home. But by August he had been shipped to England and the letters became increasingly somber. On September 8, 1918, he wrote from "somewhere in France": "I am trying to make myself as happy as I can, but it sure does go hard with me sometimes, I have the blues so bad today I can hardly write," and "you might as well let Pete have my clothes." But, returning to his optimistic tone, he assured his mother that he was "living in hope of coming back home some day." Then, the ominous passage, "but if I don't, why, we will all meet some day where we will never part." Three more short letters came from this final period, heavily censored by the chaplain. "I am praying for you mother," he wrote, "and for all the rest. I dream of being at home very often." In his last letter, September 22, 1918, he tells his mother, "I am still thinking of eating Xmas dinner at home. Don't you all worry about me." Then, almost as an afterthought: "I will meet you in heaven."

Among Uncle Dock's effects, there are five long letters from Carson Behringer, a boy from Meridian who was paralyzed from a dive into a stock tank. Though Uncle Dock's letters are never political, those from his friend are as patriotic as a recruitment poster. He wrote, "Well, Dock, this old war is a bad thing, isn't it? But let's face it brave and true and pray that it may come to a short close, but not until it can be done for the safety of righteousness

. . . and to free the world from Kaiserism, Prussianism, and Germanism and in fact everything that pertains to 'germs' and make this old world safe for democracy."

He wrote that "four airships from Waco" flew over his house and that his mother rolled him outside so that he could see them. "Oh! I would give anything," he went on, "if I could run one of them and fly over a German trench and run them Dutchmen out!"

The telegram addressed to Mrs. Sarah James advising her of the death of Andrew Jackson James came in October of 1918. The first installment check from a Bureau of War Risk Insurance policy for $10,000 arrived soon after. It was to be paid to her in installments of $57 a month. After she died, my grandmother drew it in installments of $23 a month until 1938. With these checks, my grandparents did eventually pay themselves out of debt and managed to make it through the Depression.

One of several newspaper stories describes Andrew Jackson James as one who "remained quietly within the home circle and when he did leave always accompanied the women members of the family, acquiring their gentleness and tenderness of manner."

Along with most of my mother's family, he is buried at Caddo Cemetery. On September 9, 1995, Uncle Dock and his twin sister, my grandmother, would have been 100 years old.

CHAPTER FOURTEEN

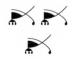

Grandpa Conner was just like Daddy and they looked as much alike as Daddy and Coon did. They had ways alike too. If they didn't like somebody they just wouldn't have anything to do with them. Grandpa Conner didn't like some of the other grandkids but he always liked you. He used to take you with him up to Bill Kelley's store and tell everybody about you. He thought everything you said was funny. One time you asked Geneva at the dinner table if you could have another biscuit because you'd run out of something to sop with. He thought that was about the funniest thing he ever heard. We thought he was old when he died but he was only eighty.

The world hasn't changed as much since 1939 as someone might think. One difference, though, is that divorce is now commonplace and sexual matters are more open. Otherwise, things are about the same. The news was filled with violence, the sordid doings of celebrity trash, racism, politics, and tragedy. "Pappy" Lee O'Daniel, a businessman with no political experience but who could sing western songs, was elected governor of Texas. W. B. Yeats, Sigmund Freud, and Supreme Court Justice Louis Brandeis died. Justice Brandeis was replaced by William O. Douglas. The Badgett quadruplets were born in Galveston.

Eleanor Roosevelt resigned from the Daughters of the American Revolution to protest that organization's refusal to allow Marian Anderson to sing at Constitution Hall. Her popularity declined even further when she publicly endorsed an anti-lynching bill in Congress. Jack Benny and George Burns were fined and placed on probation for jewel smuggling. Twenty-nine sailors died in the *Squalus* submarine tragedy. Novelist Erskine Caldwell married *Life* photographer Margaret Bourke-White.

An Alabama man traded his wife, two mules, and eighty acres for another man's young wife. Charles Lindbergh toured the country making speeches for the "Bund," said to be a pro-Hitler organization. There were bomb threats against the king and queen of England when they visited Washington. A Texas game warden was praised by the state for killing 1,165 eagles in the Big Bend area.

The chairman of the Senate Finance Committee complained of the $40 billion national debt and predicted economic chaos if the enormous federal spending is continued.

And a twenty-one-year-old, unsophisticated farm girl named Juanita Conner, who had gone to Alvin the year

before, came back to Cleburne with a month-old baby—
me. She turned me over to her parents to raise and went
back to her life at the five-and-dime, the Ace Cafe, and
Saturday nights on the town.

I enjoyed the few times with her at the ball games, an
occasional carnival, or just walking to town on Saturday
night to window-shop. Best of all, though, were the trips
with her on Sunday to spend the day with Grandpa
Conner and our two maiden aunts in Joshua. That would
be Aunt Geneva and her older sister, Aunt Harriet, my
grandfather's sisters. What a great thrill to board the big
blue and white bus in Cleburne and ride the nine miles to
Grandpa Conner's house! The bus driver was very nice
looking, and his name was Tommy. The sign on his dashboard said, "Do not talk to the operator." I didn't, but I
noticed that a lot of the women did, including my mother.
A boy looking for his real father has to suspect anyone
who has his mother's eye. And, of course, he was named
Tommy.

Grandpa Conner was the patriarch of a large family,
extending down four generations, all the way to me.
When the family gathered there on holidays, my mother
and grandmother stayed inside the house with the rest of
the women, and my grandfather and his brothers and
brothers-in-law huddled with Grandpa Conner out back
beneath the chinaberry tree to whittle and exchange stories. I was allowed to listen, but I preferred to slip away to
the shed for a secret inventory of Grandpa Conner's holdings. Horse collars and cotton scales hung on the walls,
along with farm tools and push-plows and single-tree
plows. There were iron wagon wheels for a ten-year-old
boy to roll. Barrels of corn, feed for the chickens and hogs,
were fun to thrust your hand into. Onions tied by their

blades hung from the ceiling like silver bats. An old screen door, suspended from the rafters by twine, held straight rows of red potatoes. The shed was cool inside and had a fecund aroma of life, the varied flavors of the earth. My grandfather's shed at home was similar to it, though his holdings reflected the era of the Model T instead of the horse and buggy. Raymond's was exclusively automotive and mechanical. My own "shed" is my study and my holdings are my books, archaic newspapers and magazines, manuscripts, and other reference materials.

I still have the huge rocking chair Grandpa Conner used to sit in and smoke his Prince Albert on his front porch. It looks like the chair Abraham Lincoln is sitting in at the Lincoln Memorial. When it was just the two of us, he told me fantastic tales in that same understated manner that my grandfather later perfected, whoppers calculated to send a boy into wide-eyed, heart-expanding rapture: his little dog, Judy, though she might be small, he said, was dangerous. She was a terrier dog, of a rather trepidatious disposition, I thought, but what did I know. Grandpa Conner was inerrant. "She's started going up to Joshua on a regular basis," he said, "and killing men. She brings them home and stacks them up out there in the shed. Sometimes, I sit here and watch her. She'll have one by the shirt, dragging him across the railroad tracks. They're all out there, stacked up in that shed like cordwood."

I never went back inside that shed. I eventually learned that this was where he hid his whiskey.

I sat and watched Aunt Geneva operate in her kitchen. Everything in there was military clean because, when she wasn't frying ham and making gravy and potatoes and baking bread and churning butter, she was sweeping and mopping and wiping and furiously scrubbing the walls and floors. In my kitchen stands the enormous oaken icebox that used to hold her cream and butter and eggs and everything else she wanted to keep cool. It was many years old even then. Sometimes, when I hear someone slam one of its doors and the brass handle falls hard on the latch with a loud clack! I think of her whirling about the kitchen. Her face was as bright and creamy as pie icing, without a hint of perspiration allowed to accumulate on it. Aunt Harriet was more the retiring type; she retired to the parlor to await the dinner bell. Her job was washing dishes. Her other job was to listen to everybody talk and laugh when something was funny, which was most of the time because everyone in that family was full of stories about neighbors and doings about town and anything else they could lampoon with their satirical wit.

Aunt Geneva was also the prettiest of my grandfather's sisters, I thought. Not too long ago I noticed in an old family picture that she seemed to be the only one posing. When she got old, she wore a wig. My mother said that when Aunt Geneva was young she liked boys but that Aunt Harriet seemed to be interested only in her family.

They took care of Grandpa Conner until he died in 1950. After that, Johnny Carlock, who owned the lumberyard down the road, and was a bachelor, came a-courting. He was said to be interested in both sisters but, in time, chose Aunt Geneva. What he didn't know, though, was that he also got Aunt Harriet in the bargain. Though he was otherwise notoriously tightfisted, Johnny always had a nice car, and their main entertainment was riding around and visiting relatives. Aunt Harriet was always with them. When Aunt Harriet died in 1982, they buried her on their cemetery lot in Cleburne, instead of in the family plot at Caddo.

Later, Johnny started going downhill. During my mother's residence at the retirement home, we got a call from Aunt Geneva that Uncle Johnny was "awful bad." We drove down there and were with her at her house in Joshua the night he died. She took the call, came back and sat down in her chair, brushed a tear back and said, "It's a hard old world sometimes, Nita." She wanted my mother to spend the night with her that night, but I knew that wouldn't be a good idea. She would wake up the next morning and not know where she was.

They laid Uncle Johnny to rest in the grave beside Aunt Harriet.

My mother and I visited Aunt Geneva as often as we could after that. The last time we paid her a visit at her house, my mother asked her whether she still played the piano. Yes, she said, and sent up a few bars of "The Old Rugged Cross" to prove she still had the touch. It was the same piano I used to play on as a child. It still had the same two dead keys. A few minutes after Aunt Geneva finished playing, my mother asked her, "Aunt Geneva, do you ever play the piano anymore?"

Aunt Geneva fell and broke her hip soon after that and we visited her at the hospital. "How did you break your hip, Aunt Geneva?" I said. It was almost unbelievable that this blind and toothless, withered shank of a human being was the same person as the vibrant, beautiful girl with the lively blue eyes and creamy skin that I used to watch whirling about the kitchen on those wonderful Joshua Sunday afternoons.

"Oh, Tommy," she said, disgustedly, "I got up to answer the telephone and tripped over that old pie-ana." Her mind was still fine but, like Raymond's, her body was wasted by the ravages of time.

We were surprised to learn from the doctor that she was blind. She had kept it hidden. "The Conners don't complain," my mother said. The doctor was surprised that she died so soon after that. "She seemed to give up," he said.

Someday, someone may note the three gravestones side by side on the Carlock family lot and wonder about the one that says, "Harriet Conner" and why it's there, next to that married couple. I know why and also have a pretty good idea why Aunt Geneva gave up and wouldn't eat in the nursing home. She wasn't too comfortable with Uncle Johnny and Aunt Harriet lying out there together at Rose Hill without her.

CHAPTER FIFTEEN

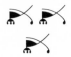

Before I went to work downtown I kept house for an old couple, way over on the other side of town, on Poindexter Street, for two and a half a week. That just barely paid for the shoes I wore out walking all the way over there and back every day. Bernice left home about that time and got a job keeping house for Dr. Porter in Fort Worth. Don't you remember her talking about Mrs. Porter? She had a cat named Fluffy. There's a picture of Fluffy in that old trunk. Then, she went to work for the bomber plant. She said she was a tailskinner. I never knew what that was. She used to let you play in her toolbox. She always said you were a pill. You were always crazy about Bernice. She met Pat in Fort Worth and they got married and moved down to the coast.

Coon was already gone by that time. He and Sarah got

*married and then he highwayed it to California and got a job
with the Southern Pacific. Not too long after that Sarah went
out there and they've been there ever since. They won't ever
come back. Durwood's buried out there.*

*Wayne joined the navy. He wasn't old enough but Daddy
signed for him to go. Wayne told him he was going to go anyway on his next birthday so Daddy just said there was nothing
he could do about it. Not too long after the war started
Wayne's ship went down and it was a long time before we knew
if he was alive or dead. Finally we heard he'd been rescued.*

*He was always a good boy. He milked cows out at
Wiseman's dairy. He got up every morning at three o'clock
and rode his bicycle all the way out there. Then, somebody
stole it. It was brand new. That was bad because he worked
hard to buy that bicycle. That really hurt Wayne. He joined
the navy right after that. Then, there was just you and me left
at home.*

At one point I thought I had it all figured out. She got
pregnant by the major league ballplayer named Tommy,
then went to Houston to an unwed mothers' home and
came back with me, a little third baseman.

"No way," said Aunt Bernice, when I told her my theory in a telephone call. All of my mother's veiled references to some scandal in her past had prompted me to ask
Aunt Bernice about it. "You can rule him out," she said.
"He's not the culprit." Aunt Bernice is as cool and logical
as my mother is dreamy and sentimental. She's also
straightforward. Growing up, I always looked to her when
I wanted the truth.

She listened to my story but said very little, other than
that I had the wrong suspect. She called back the next

morning, however. It was the most important phone call of my life. She began by saying that she didn't believe the story about A. B. Dodge either. "You don't look like him or talk like him, and you're a lot bigger. I never believed that story."

Then, she dropped the boom. She knew who my real father was!

"I never said anything till now because I was waiting for you to ask and I didn't want to interfere. Every time I thought I had my mind made up to tell you, Pat talked me out of it. He tried this time, too, but my mind was made up. He said it'll just hurt a lot of people. I said Tommy's already hurting. He deserves to know who his father is and I'm going to tell him what I think.

"I always hoped y'all would work it out. I never liked the way she just put you off on Mama and Daddy and took no responsibility for you, but I didn't think it was my place to say anything."

This is what she told me:

"When we lived over there on East James your mother used to spend a lot of time visiting with the Manns, who lived in an apartment right behind us. They moved down to Alvin in 1937 or '38, and it wasn't too long after that Nita left home and went to Alvin, too. The next thing I knew she had you.

"A few years later she came down to visit us in La Porte and she hadn't been there very long before Clarence Mann showed up. I was surprised to see him because I hadn't heard from him since I left Cleburne. Then, all of a sudden, he just showed up at my house. And I thought at the time that they had something going. You can just tell. The way they were acting was just like, well, they were more than friends. Now, why in the world did he show up that day at my house? How did he know where I lived? The only answer is that she called him and told him she was going to be there. That's the only thing it could have been. I believe that Clarence Mann is your father. The first time I ever saw you I thought you looked just like him. And the older you got the more you favored him. He was big like you and dark complected. I never thought you looked like Lonnie.

"And, then, there's another thing. One time when I was back home visiting, y'all had moved over to English Street by this time, Corine and her two children came by. That was Clarence's wife. They stayed around a while and she seemed awfully interested in you. I believe she just wanted to see you. Maybe she had heard something and just wanted to see what you looked like. I don't know. It may be just my imagination, but that's what I believe."

A check through the Cleburne city directories showed that Clarence Mann lived in Cleburne from 1924 through 1926, worked for the Santa Fe Railroad as a switchman and lived at various addresses. Unfortunately, the library doesn't have the directories from 1927 through 1938. But the directory for 1939, which is there, didn't list him, which backed up part of Aunt Bernice's story. Many telephone calls to Alvin turned up nothing. He was probably dead now, but his children, Jack and Helen, might be alive and in their late fifties or early sixties. Could I be their half brother?

Arrangements to have Aunt Bernice come up for a visit could never be worked out. Uncle Pat's health was failing and his hearing gone. They won't fly, and she was reluctant to drive the 250 miles with him or leave him alone at home. So, on a weekend in August 1994, I bought my mother a round-trip ticket and flew her down

there. It was a great risk, but she wanted to go. At the airport I alerted the flight attendants to her condition, and I
was allowed to see her to her seat on the plane.

"Oh, I'm so happy!" she told me. "I could never have
done this without you!"

Nice to hear, but I wish she could admit that there is
hardly anything that she can do without me. The need for
independence is strong in everyone but, someday, when
the time comes, I hope I'm able to say to anyone
approaching me with business on their minds, these simple words: "You'll have to talk to my children about this
matter. They handle all my affairs now." At the retirement home where she lives, many of the women told me,
"I was no longer able to cook and do housework, so my
children thought it best that I move out here." My mother
could as easily have flown that plane to Houston as she
could prepare a meal, do housework, shop for groceries, or
drive a car, yet she never tired of touting her expertise in
these matters to me or anyone else willing to listen. To
those who didn't know her, I then felt obliged to justify
everything I did for her.

The trip turned out to be a failure, as things almost
invariably do when undertaken with ulterior motives. I
had hoped that Aunt Bernice would do my work for me,
get my mother to open up and tell the secrets she had
kept all these years. It turned out, though, that my mother
had motives of her own. She hoped to enlist Aunt
Bernice in her relentless campaign to go back to her old
house in Cleburne. On the phone Aunt Bernice said she
just didn't think the time or setting was right to bring this
matter up. And, besides, she said, "I don't know what in
the world you're going to do with her. She can't remember anything!"

"Until you're with her for a day or two," I told her, "you just don't know how bad it really is. Now you know."

"All she wanted to talk about was Mama and Daddy and Raymond. And she worked on me the whole time to help her persuade you to let her go back to Cleburne. I told her over and over that she ought to shut up about Cleburne, that Raymond and Mama and Daddy are dead, and she ought to admit that and quit trying to act like they weren't. 'You can't live with the dead,' I told her. I said, 'That's what's the matter with your mind, now. You keep everything inside of you just like Mama did. You won't tell anybody and it all builds up inside you. You just can't do that without it taking its toll on you. If you have something to tell to Tommy, then you need to do it.' I was pretty hard on her, but she took it and didn't start up with those tears. I thought she would but she didn't. She wouldn't open up, and so I decided this wasn't the time. I let it go. She just wanted to talk about getting back to Cleburne.

"She knew how I felt about that, so when I would doze off, she'd start in on Pat, trying to get him on her side. But he told her the same thing. So she didn't get much sympathy out of us."

Then Aunt Bernice told me all the peculiar things my mother did:

"She couldn't remember which bedroom was hers."

"She hid my massager under her pillow."

"Every time she asked if I had heard from Wayne I had to tell her that he had a stroke. Then she was upset every time I told her."

"Before we could leave for the airport we had to hunt for her purse. I found it in my closet hidden behind some clothes."

"If she told me once she told me a thousand times that you were supposed to come and pick her up."

This litany of my mother's doings was all too familiar to me but shocking and bewildering to the uninitiated. Waiting for her at the airport, I questioned my decision to send her alone on this trip. She clearly needed someone with her, though flight attendants are accustomed to travelers like her. If the trip hadn't suited my purposes, would I have sent her? Was it too much an inconvenience for Aunt Bernice? Or too painfully sad for her to see how the disease had done its damage? Would my mother even remember that she went?

No to the last question.

She looked panicky as she came off the plane. An attendant walked beside her carrying her bag. They were both relieved to see me. "I'm so glad you're here," the attendant said. Then, she tried to tell me something that had happened on the plane but was reluctant to do so with my mother standing beside her. Whatever it was, I didn't want to know at the time.

"How did you know to be here?" my mother asked me.

"Well, I told you I'd be here to pick you up and take you home. Bernice would put you on the plane in Houston and I'd meet you in Dallas."

During the long walk to the car, she said, "I made a boo-boo on the plane."

No amount of interrogation could get to the bottom of it, however. All she said was, "Don't tell anybody I made a boo-boo on the plane."

I said I wouldn't because I wasn't there and didn't know what she did. I called the airline several times but never found out.

"Just don't tell anybody I had a bad flight."

I told her that any flight that doesn't crash is a good flight, in my opinion.

"How did the plane stop?" she asked me.

I think she meant how did the pilot know to take her to where I was and let her off? But I didn't pursue it. I had more important ground to cover.

"I'd rather talk about Clarence Mann," I said, as we headed south toward home.

"He's dead," she said, obviously surprised.

"How do you know that?"

"He was old."

"He had a son named Jack and a daughter named Helen."

An old intensity suddenly replaced the usual dormant look on her face. "How did you know that?" she said.

"Bernice told me."

She thought about this for a moment. "His wife was named Corine."

"What about her?"

"She's dead, too."

"Tell me about him."

"He drank a lot." She said this very softly, under her breath almost. This was all I was going to get out of her. So I let it go for now.

Before we got home, she was talking about her bus ride. She had forgotten where she went and that she had gone on a plane.

More disappointing to me, the mystery of my birth was still locked in her ever-narrowing memory. That night, I had the dream again about the old trunk and the key inside it that I was blamed for losing.

CHAPTER SIXTEEN

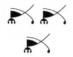

W e were living at Egan,
way out in the sticks, when I was born. That would be 1918.
I may forget how old I am but I always know when I was born.
Mama always said those were the hardest times of her life, way
out there in the brush. She was just about twenty-three years
old when the baby died with the pneumonia. Daddy had the
typhoid fever. Uncle Dock left for the war. Coon was three
and I was just a month old when the baby died.

It took old Dr. Pearson the longest time to get out there from
Joshua in a buggy when the baby died. Daddy was still sick but
he walked up to the Galts' house and used the telephone to call
him. Egan had telephones back then. Mama used to say it was
a big city in those days. It had two grocery stores and a general
store. A broom factory. A Methodist church. A lodge hall of

some kind. A drugstore. Cotton gin, barber shop, produce market, railroad, you name it. It even had a place where they made wine. A man named Martin made wine and sold it to all the railroad workers, they say, and I guess, anybody else that wanted it. There was a school there with fifty or sixty kids in it. I don't know if we were there when Coon started to school or not. If he did, I pity the schoolteacher.

Mama said she just had to leave me on the bed by myself while Howard was burning up with fever. He was just sixteen months old when he died. Daddy borrowed $5 from Grandpa Conner and bought that cemetery lot out at Caddo. He paid him back in oats. Now they're all buried out there, even Raymond. I wish I was too.

On the day after my mother's return from Houston I got a call from Aunt Bernice saying that a five-by-seven framed picture of my grandparents was missing, that she had called my mother, who had denied taking it or even having any knowledge of it. I told her I would go over and look for the picture. Lindon was visiting us, and he went along just to say hello.

The picture was sitting on her dresser. I put it in my pocket and started to leave when she brought up her usual topic: when would she get to go back to her house in Cleburne? "Oh, why can't I just die?" she moaned. "Oh, nobody knows! Nobody knows!"

Everything came crashing down on me at that moment —the trip's failure to turn up anything new, her continual stonewalling, her inability to appreciate Lindon's visit without involving him in her campaign to get back to Cleburne. It seemed that blocking me at every turn was her mission in life. I blew up and stomped out of the house. "Lindon just came over for a visit," I told her. "Why can't you just appreciate that? Instead you have to bring up this same old refrain! About how you want to die, how you want to move back to Cleburne. I'm getting sick of it!"

She followed me into the yard. "Tommy," she said, "don't fuss at me. I just wonder about things," she said. "I wonder if somebody is living in my house. I wonder about my money in the bank. Things like that." I decided then that if she could bring up moving to Cleburne every time she saw me, then I had the right to bring up my own question. So, I said it:

"Well, I wonder about things, too. Do you want to hear what I wonder about? Do you? Well, I'll tell you. I wonder about who my real father was. That's what I wonder about!"

She shushed me. "The neighbors will have the police on us!" she said.

"It isn't a crime to ask your mother who your father was!" I said. This came from resentment built up from many years of silence. Then, I let it all go. How I felt. All of it. Even the humiliation of having to fill out forms in school and not knowing what to put in the blank asking for your father's name. Maybe I couldn't have done it if Lindon hadn't been there to support me. "I want to know, once and for all," I said. "Who was my real father?"

"Your daddy was Lonnie Dodge!" she said, without hesitating. It seemed like an all-too-familiar script, a little too easy. More likely, a last-ditch attempt to hide the truth. "I want to hear the whole story," I said.

She promised to tell me everything. Right then, she said, she couldn't remember it all. She would tell me tomorrow.

It was a mixed victory. I had at least brought it out into the open, but I had been angry and, I felt, too hard on her. But Aunt Bernice had told me that you can't be easy with her because she can manipulate you with her tears and her *Exorcist* impersonation. So, I guess I did what had to be done at the time.

"I'm sorry I acted that way," she said as we were leaving. "Will you come back to see me, Lindon?"

"I'll come back," he said. "But I don't ever want to hear you say you want to die again."

"I'm sorry. I know how you suffer and I shouldn't say things like that to you. All I want is to go back to Cleburne. If I can go back to Cleburne I won't ever bother anybody again. I promise."

"All right," I said. "You pick out the doctor of your choice and I'll take you to see him for a test. If he says you're able to live on your own, then that's what I'll abide by. But if he says you can't, then you have to shut up about living in Cleburne by yourself and let me take care of you."

"I'll sure do that!" she said. "I can still cook and clean house. And I can drive, too. You just give me a chance and I'll show you."

A day or two later I took some of the A. B. Dodge memorabilia over to her house and showed it all to her. His letters and photographs especially interested her. She looked it all over and asked if I had any more. I asked her what happened to the trove of German jewelry and medals that she used to have. "That I couldn't tell you," she said. She could remember the names of everybody who lived in our neighborhood and everybody on both sides of East Henderson Street in the 1940s, but she couldn't remember what happened to an entire box of valuable jewelry.

One week later, August 6, 1994, I tried again. With just the two of us, in her living room, I showed her the material again. I told her that I was going to read from one of the letters and it might be upsetting to her but that I had to do it.

She said, "Don't do it if it's going to be bad."

"I didn't say it would be bad. To me it isn't bad. I said it might be upsetting." Then, I took out the letter written to me from A. B. Dodge when I lived in Brenham in 1969. I read it out loud: "You were born in a home for unwed mothers in Houston. Your mother brought you to see me when you were one week old and said I was your father. So I paid for your keep for a while, but then she said she didn't want to get married and wanted to move back and stay with her parents in Cleburne. You might have heard of Clarence Mann. I kept up with you through him."

All my life I had fantasized about this moment, whether it would ever happen. If it did, how would she react? Would she collapse in a tearful, guilt-inducing histrionic heap? It seemed unreal that I was actually doing it, and her reaction was nothing like I thought it would be. In fact, she listened calmly, without tears this time. "So what does this mean?" I asked. "'I kept up with you through Clarence Mann.' Who was Clarence Mann?"

Though confronting her was much easier than I thought it would be, I still felt guilty doing it. She suffers over the smallest of problems. Thinking she might never find the TV clicker can bring real tears. I was probing into a sore spot that had ached inside her heart for fifty-five years. She rocked gently in her chair. "He was a friend of ours," she said. "His wife was named Corine. They lived behind us. The Hubbards lived on the corner. His wife was named Corine. They had a daughter named Helen and a boy named Jack."

I told her Aunt Bernice's story about Clarence Mann showing up at her house that time. "She said there was no way he could have known where she lived if you hadn't told him. She said she could tell then there was something between the two of you."

"I don't remember that," she said. She was still looking at the keepsakes. An old issue of *Stars and Stripes* turned yellow with age caught her eye. She had just come back from the beauty shop. She looked twenty years younger than her age.

"Bernice says you left Cleburne and went to Alvin in 1938. Why did you do that? Of all the towns to move to, why Alvin?"

"I don't remember that. Let me think about it and I'll tell you tomorrow."

"No. You won't. You won't bring it up, and I don't know if I'll be able to, either. You need to tell me now. Look. Don't worry about what I'm going to think. I'll be fine. And you will be, too. Didn't Bernice tell you that she thought your mind is going bad because you keep all these things to yourself? Don't you think you'll feel better about it if you tell me and get it out in the open? I promise you I won't hold it against you—whatever it is. Whatever happened was a long time ago. You were young. You did the best you could. Nobody's going to judge you."

She rocked and looked at the *Stars and Stripes*. "People like to gossip about you. It's better to keep secrets. I'm like Mama. She kept everything, too."

"People who care about you won't hold it against you. They know you're a good person. Everybody makes mistakes. Forget what other people think. The good people won't hold it against you, and the ones that do aren't worth caring about."

She began to cry softly, but she was calm.

"I have all these letters and things from A. B. Dodge," I said. "All he said was that you said he was my father. He never said he was. I never thought I looked like him. Do you think I do?"

"No, you don't."

"Why not?"

"I don't know."

"Do I look like Clarence Mann?"

"Yes."

"Why do I look like Clarence Mann?"

"I don't know."

"Tell me about him."

"He had a wife named Corine. They lived behind us on James Street. The Hubbards lived on the corner."

"I'm not interested in his wife or the neighbors. I want to know about him."

"He was tall. And big. He drank a lot."

"Tell me why you moved to Alvin. Was it because the Manns moved down there, and you followed them because you were involved with him?"

"I went down there to work. I got a job in a dime store."

"Where did you live?"

She stalled again. "I don't remember much of that. I'll have to think about it. Let me sleep on it and I'll tell you all of it tomorrow."

"How come you can remember everything else that happened in those days but you can't remember this?"

"I guess I just skipped it out of my mind."

"Do you want to know what Bernice thinks?"

"Yes."

"She thinks that you got involved with Clarence Mann and I came along as a result. Since he was married you just gave me the name of another man you were involved with because he was single. And that would also explain why you didn't want to marry A. B. Dodge."

"I don't remember." She looked through the double doors into the backyard. "Tipper knows you're in here. Sometimes I see him running around the house so he can look across the street to see if your truck is there. He's got a trail worn out where he runs back and forth." She picked up the daily paper, looked at it, then tossed it aside. Its banner headlines included health care, the Whitewater scandal, and the O. J. Simpson murder trial. "I wish they'd stop throwing that paper. There's never anything in it. Newspapers aren't any good till they're yellow."

She began to cry softly again. "I just did the best I could," she said. "I brought you back home when you were six weeks old and went to work. We all took care of you. I worked and bought you things. Mama made your clothes. You had what you needed. I always thought you were happy. I didn't know what else to do. I know I should have told you, and I wish I had. But I didn't. I just didn't want anybody to know it."

"Did Ann-A know the story?"

"She knew. But she didn't talk about it. I learned how to keep secrets like she did."

I wanted to hug her and comfort her, but years of education in the art of restraint had done their work. Instead, I said, "It's all right. Times have changed. Nobody cares anymore. I certainly don't hold it against you. I'm a long way from being perfect myself. And I'm grateful that you didn't give me up to be adopted."

"That never entered my mind. I knew we could raise you."

"I just wish you hadn't worried so much about what people thought. Are you still worried about it?"

"It'll just give the old ladies something else to talk about."

"They're just jealous of you because you don't have any gray hair and look a lot younger than they do. Don't worry about what they think. People that gossip have empty lives."

"Do you think my hair looks good? I washed it and rolled it up today."

"I think it looks great. Did you have a good time at Bernice's?"

She strained to remember. "Yes," she said. "It was a long bus ride, though. Next time I'm going to ride the train. Mama and Daddy used to ride the train all the time. Daddy loved to ride the train. He always took you along. Y'all rode it to California to see Coon and Sarah. Do you remember that?"

"I remember."

"Those were good days. Not like now."

We didn't say anything for a while. She looked up when the clocks struck four. The mantel clock struck a few seconds ahead of the one on the wall. "The wall clock runs slow," she said. "Raymond had them where they'd strike together." She looked into the hall. "Where's Maudie?" she said.

"Maudie went home for the weekend. She'll be back at six."

"She will?"

"Yes. She goes home on Thursday and comes back on Saturday."

"Maudie's a good cook. She cooks like Mama used to. She gets up in the morning before I do and fixes my breakfast and my coffee. I wait on her till she gets hers fixed and then we eat. Maudie's a good person. But I don't think she likes me."

"You never did say anything about what Bernice believes happened. That you followed the Manns to Alvin and had me and gave me A.B. Dodge's name because he was single."

"I'll think about that and tell you tomorrow."

"It's real simple. Either it's true or it isn't. All you have to say is —"

"Yes or no."

"Right. All I want to know is — who was my real father?"

She looked outside through the glass door. Tipper was lying against it, slowly and thoughtfully scratching his ear. She started to say something, then stopped and picked up the newspaper again and laid it back down. Then, her mouth formed the words and I seemed to hear them strangely out of sync, like a character in a foreign movie with another language dubbed in:

"It was Clarence Mann."

CHAPTER SEVENTEEN

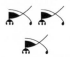

Oh, lord, with all the hardships Mama had to suffer, I wonder how she stood up. The baby dying, Uncle Dock getting killed, living on those old wore-out sandy-land farms, having to carry water, Grandma James losing her mind. And, oh, how she suffered with the asthma like she did and with the dropsy, too. The doctor told her that if she didn't have an operation on her heart that she was going to die. She said she wasn't going to let them cut on her. Daddy didn't want the doctors to cut on her, either. He said they cut on Grandpa Conner and killed him. So, she wouldn't do it. She believed that when it was your time to go then that was it. I guess she was right because she got over it somehow. I used to wonder how she did it but she just said the good lord won't ever put more on you than you can take. I *guess that's right, but with her, it looked like the good lord was trying to see how much she could take.*

And so we had traveled together across Lethe's Plain, through thunder and lightning, back like shooting stars to the time of my birth. And for her, I think, finally, all was well.

As for me, finding out that my father was someone other than the one I had thought was harder to accept than I believed it would be. My mind racing, my heart pounding in my chest, and a muscle spasm in my left leg kept me awake all night. The next afternoon Lindon brought me some Valium, which quickly gave me some relief.

Nothing could keep me from digging even deeper into this family secret. Just as I had searched out A. B. Dodge in 1968, I was determined to do the same for the family of Clarence Mann. It had become an obsession with me to find that mysterious and unique someone with whom I share a likeness that originates deep inside the DNA of fathers, the chromosome that slides down the curvature of the double helix and stamps its family seal on a succession of descendants. Finding such a link would, I believed, relieve the dark, abiding feeling of loneliness and alienation I have felt all my life.

I have never envied anyone else's possessions. I envy their physical and spiritual bond with their father and their brothers and sisters. It is literally a painful feeling not to have a father. My sons are comforted to see the source of their looks, movements, and voice tones in me. Sometimes, when Lowell calls, his mother mistakes him for me. She used to say that Lindon walked exactly like me. I always wanted to see that in a father. My grandfather was a great man; his upright behavior was exemplary in the eyes of his many friends, and his world view was Taoistic in its harmonious simplicity. I'm grateful for the influence he had on me. But it just wasn't the same. He was the father of Coon and Wayne, his own sons. Raymond was the most intelligent, kindest, most even-tempered man I ever knew, but he wasn't my father. The worst day of the year for me was Father's Day. I resented it and refused to acknowledge it. Maybe I should have bought my grandfather or Raymond a card, but I never did. It was my way of protesting.

I have some qualities, good and bad, that are distinctly different from those of the Conner family. This was one reason I have always been obsessed with finding my true father. That he apparently made no effort to find me bothered me, but maybe there was some explanation for it. Maybe he did keep up with me and my doings, as the letter said. The image of someone watching me secretly in the background as I played baseball, sang in school plays, graduated from college — this was an appealing fantasy, and could have happened. If someone was watching, he never let me know, never contacted me. I realized that he was probably dead now. He would be over ninety years old.

I visited my mother the next day. She was all right. As far as I knew, she had re-immersed herself in the healing waters of Lethe. We talked about other things, the dog, mainly, and his doings. I gave her all the A B. Dodge memorabilia, then reconsidered and took it back before it disappeared forever into the black hole. Someday, I would probably give it back to "Aunt" Edith. I still have an affection for the memory of the man A. B. Dodge, who was so happy that I contacted him with the news that I was his son. He wrote that he had always told people he had a son, but he was afraid no one believed him. I sent him photos of my family, and when he was killed in a car crash in 1971, the framed pictures were part of his few personal effects. From all I have learned, he was a sincere, happy-go-lucky man who happened also to be something of a "rounder," especially when it came to women. He said in a letter that he had always been "poor but honest and hard working." He was proud of his war record, and he was proud of me and proud that he could finally prove to others that he did, in fact, have a family somewhere.

I have developed over the years an affectionate relationship with Aunt Edith, who will, I hope, always regard me as her nephew. She is an intelligent, beautiful woman in her eighties who lives in Brazoria, near the Texas Gulf Coast. We visit sometimes on the telephone, and she always signs off with "I love you, Tommy Ray!" I have met her daughter, Carolyn, and her family, and we keep in touch. Each Christmas she sends me a detailed account of her year's doings. I have met my Aunt Lucy in Texarkana, who graciously supplied me with a trove of photos of A. B. Dodge. I viewed them as family. There is no reason as far as I am concerned for our relationship to change.

There doesn't seem to be a word in the language that defines the emotion I felt that Sunday my mother told me the truth. What is the word for someone who invests a lifetime in associating himself with a family that turns out to be the wrong family? Sucker is much too general. Dupe? This fits but, again, too general. I even spent time one summer researching the Dodge family back to 1810. I joined the Dodge Family Association and bought all the Dodge family history books. Now, it was time to switch families, which presented another problem: what if I meet them and they reject me? What if I resemble them physically but am radically different from them spiritually and in every other meaningful way?

I wanted to tell my mother again that I was glad she kept me instead of giving me up to be adopted, that by doing this she gave me a great gift. But I had done that already and didn't want to rekindle any of the burning pain she might have forgotten. I hope this book doesn't do that, either. She and I differ, obviously, on the importance of keeping this secret. Her way of handling it hasn't worked. I believe, as George Bernard Shaw has said, that you can't hide a family skeleton in the closet forever, so you might as well take it out and make it dance.

CHAPTER EIGHTEEN

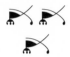

Coon always looked just like Daddy. They were a lot alike in their ways, too. That's why they didn't always get along. Daddy was always whipping him for something or other. Usually, he deserved it, he was so mean. One time, Daddy heard him cussing when he didn't think anybody was around. He was trying to fix something, a harness or something. He was just cussing a blue streak, and Daddy walked up. I think Coon must have told Daddy he'd cuss all he wanted to, or something like that. Boy, Daddy let him have it with his belt like you wouldn't believe. Daddy never allowed any cussing. He didn't do it hisself. But they were both stubborn. That's the main way they were alike in ways. When Coon got grown, he looked just like Daddy — and he stopped cussing.

Mama always believed in blood. She didn't believe in adopting. "Blood is thicker than water" — I've heard her say that a million times.

On Wednesday, August 10, 1994, I placed the following ad in the personal section of the Alvin newspaper: "Information wanted on the whereabouts of the family of Clarence Mann." A few days later, there was a recording on my answering machine from Barbara Quinn, who told me that she was the daughter of Helen Mann Hollingsworth and that Clarence Mann was her grandfather. She didn't leave her telephone number, and I was afraid I wouldn't hear from her again.

But she called back that same evening with the information that she and her mother, who had recently been diagnosed with terminal cancer, had been living in the East Texas town of Henderson for two years. Her Uncle Jack, she said, lived on a farm in Angleton, near the Texas coast. But her reason for calling was curiosity: why did I want to contact them?

I was looking for information about my father, I told her, and in one of his letters he had written that he had kept up with me through a friend, Clarence Mann. She was open and cordial from the first. She said that her grandfather died in 1972, of an aneurysm, at the age of sixty-nine. He and her grandmother had owned and operated a bar and grill for many years before retiring. Her grandmother died in the 1980s. She said she asked her mother but she hadn't remembered me. I told her I wasn't born when my family and hers were neighbors.

I would like to talk with her uncle, I said, and she told me she would write or call back with his telephone number. She seemed surprised when I reminded her that she had failed to leave her telephone number on my answering machine, but she still didn't volunteer it.

A week passed and I didn't hear from her. I wished I had pointedly asked for her number, as I had found through information that there were no Henderson listings for her or her mother. Jack Mann's number in Angleton was unpublished. A call to the Henderson library turned up no listing in the city directory for her or her mother, but the librarian was able to find Barbara's number in the Rusk County telephone directory.

I called and left a message that I would like to speak with her again. She didn't return the call, so I called again that evening, and she answered. Making this call was an extraordinary thing for me. Ordinarily, persistence isn't one of my strong characteristics. I assume that when a call isn't returned within a reasonable length of time I am being told to take a long walk on a short pier. Whenever I'm tempted to persist in matters, there is a voice inside of me saying, "A real man never begs." But, actually, testosterone has nothing to do with it. It is the result of a long-held fear of being unwanted, a fear that exacts a heavy toll over a lifetime. This time, though, I made the call.

As any rational person would have expected, it was only a miscommunication. She was happy I had called, and we chatted about her family. At this time she said that her mother did, in fact, remember my mother and Aunt Bernice. "What was your father's name?" she asked.

I told her A. B. (Lonnie) Dodge, and she said that she remembered him very well from childhood, that he had worked at a grocery store in Alvin in the early 1950s near where she lived. She said that her mother had now remembered my mother. "Your mother had an affair with

Lonnie, and she got pregnant and they never got married," Barbara said. "Is that right?"

"That's what I was told," I said. Then, I said I would like to meet her and her mother if it would be all right and wouldn't upset her mother in any way. She was willing to do this and we set up a time for the following Sunday afternoon.

A few minutes later she called back. "You might think I'm crazy," she said, "but I have to ask this question."

I said that would be fine. I really had no idea what she was going to ask.

"You wouldn't be interested in our family because you might have some idea that my grandfather was your father?" she said.

This took me by surprise. All I could think of to say was, "What makes you think that?"

"It was the questions you asked," she said, "about my grandfather and when he died, how old he was and what was wrong with him."

I still couldn't forge the courage to tell her the truth. So, I stammered some more.

"If you do think that, I want you to know that I'm not bothered by it," she said. "After all these years, it wouldn't bother me if it were true."

I was relieved and decided that Mark Twain was right: when in doubt, tell the truth. "I'll be honest with you," I said. "I've always been puzzled by that remark in a letter from A. B. Dodge that your grandfather had kept up with me and my activities as I was growing up. Then, a while back, my Aunt Bernice told me she thought Clarence Mann was my real father. I was hesitant to tell you this because I was afraid of being rejected. This is very impor-

tant to me, and I didn't want to take any chances. I
wanted to meet you first."

"It's no secret in our family that my grandfather was
a womanizer," she said. "My mother told me this and
said that it almost caused a divorce. If you are his son, I
wouldn't be surprised—or bothered by it. And I don't
think my mother would be, either." She went on to say
that she would discuss it with her mother but again
assured me that our visit wouldn't be jeopardized by the
discussion. I asked her to hold off telling her, and she said
she would until after she had talked with her sister, Janet,
who was staying with Helen.

The day before my trip to Henderson was bleak and
achingly solitary, one in which I felt helpless to clear the
murky clouds from my brain. I was entangled in a web of
undefinable emotion. A protective wall that had taken a
lifetime to build was crumbling around me, leaving me
vulnerable, scared, and almost inert. I greatly needed to
reach out to someone but was unable to do it. Later, when
I complained that no one offered me any comfort, someone told me, "You won't let anybody."

The answer to the central question of my life was now
within reach, just a short three-hour drive away, and I was
seized up like a blown engine. My thoughts lurched about
incoherently. All alone I sat inside all day, seeing no one,
speaking to no one, most of the time unable to connect
two rational thoughts together. From time to time, I managed to shift from my chair to the sofa, staring dully at the
television screen for hours. My emotional configuration
was so skewed that I could neither smile nor cry. I imagined that my face had caved in like a poorly prepared
cake. How emotionally fragile we humans are! There is

nothing so good that happens to us that we can't agonize over it.

Though I had planned to get an early start the next morning, I stalled till the last minute. Finally getting underway, I took several wrong turns. It looked as though I would be late, but on Sunday morning the freeway was almost empty and I found myself driving eighty on the interstate. A *Prairie Home Companion* was playing on the radio. Garrison Keillor's droll stories and wit lifted my spirits until, near the end of the show, he sang "Amazing Grace." I pretended that he was singing to me, that he knew what I was going through, and he was singing this wonderfully redeeming song for me. I finally began to cry as the emotion of these lines washed over me:

> Amazing grace! how sweet the sound
> That saved a wretch like me!
> I once was lost, but now am found,
> Was blind but now I see.

I could see a change in the terrain as I left the bare and muted landscape of Dallas County behind and crossed over into East Texas. Both sides of the highway were lined with pines, pin oaks, red oaks, live oaks, and dogwoods, so high they blocked the morning sun. I turned off the air conditioner and lowered the windows. The lush fragrances awakened my dull spirit and lifted my expectations. It was only a matter of minutes now. A word of revelation from my aunt, a brief ad in a small newspaper, a single call from only one reader in Alvin to a relative in Henderson: it had all come down to this moment as I stopped my car in the driveway of Barbara and Charles Quinn.

Barbara has dark hair and light green eyes and looks

and moves amazingly like our daughter Karen. She smiled and extended her hand in welcome. Her husband is a rugged cowboy, a prize-winning team roper. They live on thirty-seven acres in a picturesque log house decorated in a western motif.

They stared at me intently.

She introduced me to her sister, Janet Hutton, also a brunette with green eyes and a warm smile, and to Barbara's daughter, Darla. Darla held her small baby. I could feel their eyes drilling into me. Even the baby couldn't take its eyes off of me. "There's no doubt," Janet said. "He looks just like Granddaddy. Especially from the side, when he turns his head, and through the eyes and forehead." Charles agreed.

Barbara kept staring, with a kind of stunned reluctant certainty in her face.

They listened interestedly as I told my story, then Barbara brought out the family photo albums.

Darla's husband, Steven, came in the back door as I opened the albums, and I heard her tell him, "He looks just like Uncle Jack."

I gazed down into the photographs and, for the first time in my life, saw the likeness of my true father. Here he was, this mystery man who suddenly seemed not so mysterious at all—a darkly handsome guy in a tough, underworldly way, about six feet tall, 180 pounds, dark receding hair, and heavy eyebrows. He stands beside a 1934 Ford roadster with his Stetson in his hand. He is clearly uncomfortable with all this picture-taking but is accommodating the woman with the camera. We gaze at one another across the rubble of broken hearts, spent emotion, gossip real and imagined, lies told and untold, desperate childhood fantasies, and family secrets.

I see it all in his iron face, in his not-quite-sincere smile. He wears his secret uneasily, like a shirt a half-size too small. He looks distrustfully into the camera, as if the lens might tell too much. He folds his arms across his chest, like a rugged Dimmesdale forever clutching his heart.

I stared at the photos of my new half brother, Jack. He, too, has the unmistakable stamp of sad amiability in his eyes. Helen, as a teenager, looks enough like Karen to be her sister.

It was Janet who urged her sister to call Helen. "There's no doubt in my mind," she said again. "Despite the long hair, the beard, and the glasses, it's unmistakable. There's just no doubt. Oh, my word! Just look at him from the side when he turns his head! It's just like Granddaddy! I know Mother would be happy to see him." Janet and I felt an immediate closeness. She had listened with great interest when I had tried to convey my ambiguous feelings about being relegated as a child to the care of my grandparents. She said she had felt much the same ambiguity growing up, as she, too, had been raised by her grandparents.

"Mama said to come on over. She wants to see you," Barbara told me.

I was hesitant. I didn't want to upset her.

"Oh, you won't," she said. "She'll be fine."

"As long as you don't say anything nice about the Republicans," Charles said. Spoken like a true son-in-law. We chuckled.

Janet's early reluctance to bring Helen and me together was based on her mother's illness. Helen was swollen from the seventeen kinds of medication she had been taking, and she had lost her hair from radiation treatments,

treatments she had recently ordered halted because of the pain and debilitation. In effect, she said she preferred three good months to a year of misery.

"She hates for you to see her this way," Janet told me. "Just last May she was fit as a fiddle. Now, she doesn't look like herself." The women explained that we would give her time to get herself "fixed up" and then drive the nine miles to her home. It was a "female thing."

Helen met me at the door with great affection and enthusiasm. She studied me and smiled broadly.

"What do you think, Mother?" one of the sisters asked.

"Oh, there's no doubt," she said immediately. "I wasn't a bit surprised to hear about you, Tom," she went on. "Daddy was . . . well, let's just say that the women liked him, and he didn't exactly try to fight them off. So, no, I'm not at all surprised to hear about you."

Our visit consisted of more family history, more photographs, more revelation. After a while, Helen said, "I knew about Daddy and Nita. She lived in the house with us when she came to Alvin. My mother worked and Nita didn't, and one day I came home from school early and caught them together. I told Mother about it and that's when Nita left. But I guess the damage had already been done."

I was the damage, I thought. I was my mother's scarlet letter that she refused to wear. I had been, instead, just a constant reminder of her folly. When Raymond died, the women at her church had never known my last name.

"She must have had an affair with Lonnie, too, but I know he was also going with a beauty operator in town named Merle. He was a rounder, too."

We looked at pictures some more, and they urged me to select some. They would have them copied and sent to me. Helen said she would call Jack that evening. He won't be surprised, she told me. "Somebody told him a long time ago that he had a double living in Cleburne." This somebody, she thought, was W. D. "Dub" Booth, Clarence's half brother.

It had been a tender and happy meeting for us all. Leaving, embraces replaced handshakes, and when Helen took me in her arms, tears became involved. "I hope I live long enough to read your book," she said.

The suddenness and shock of seeing a sister I never knew I had and knowing that our time to spend together was limited to a matter of months, maybe weeks or days, seeing pictures of a father I never knew I had, evoked such complicated and unfamiliar emotions in me, that my life-long feeling that I was a stranger to my own self seemed compounded. Janet followed me outside to my car and comforted me. "It's too bad that I was almost too late," I managed to say.

"You'll still have Jack," she said. "And us."

I called Jack two days later. By telephone isn't the best way to become acquainted with someone purporting to be your long-lost brother and, though he was polite, he was obviously operating under considerable difficulty. He seemed to choose his words carefully and, I thought, with an almost legal precision. He spoke with a powerful and authoritative voice.

"Now," he said, "after all your research and whatnot, do you have any doubts about what you've found out about Clarence and Nita and that this situation is what you think it is?"

"No, she told me it was the truth."

"She actually 'fessed up, did she?"

"Yes."

"Your life, then," he said after a short pause, "growing up in that manner has, quite naturally, been somewhat hard for you. All that has happened has been, well, let's say it's been quite something else."

"Well, I guess you could put it that way. It wasn't unbearable, but it wasn't exactly very pleasant, either. It was kind of like being a stranger to one side of yourself."

"To be sure," he said, "to be sure."

After a while, he seemed to warm up. He said he had always wanted a brother and, "lo and behold," he'd had one all the time. He kept returning to his interest in my current state of mind and how I was feeling, in light of all these revelations. I must have felt I had lived my life in a "quandary," he said, but must feel somewhat relieved finally to have gotten to the bottom of it.

He told me about our father, saying that they had always been best friends and did everything together, especially hunting and fishing, but their main pastime had been arguing. His emphasis on arguing was evidently supposed to define, with extreme clarity, the tight bond between them, as he went on to say, "Anybody will tell you that I'm pretty damned particular who I argue with."

He seemed interested that I thought I resembled both him and "Clarence," because he said he never thought he looked like his father. He told me the story of how Clarence's father, Sam Houston Mann, had left Cleburne for parts unknown before Clarence was born, under great duress. Clarence never met him or knew what happened to him. All Jack ever heard him say about it was that if his father was across the street, he wouldn't walk across to see him. This incident turned out to be another great family secret. Apparently, Miss Tula May Pollock, in her teens and impressionable, encountered this handsome, older man, maybe an itinerant railroad worker, and nature took over. Later, I located the marriage certificate in the Johnson County courthouse, dated May 13, 1901. Evidently, shotguns had been involved, and Sam Houston Mann vanished. Maybe he died due to one of her father's or brothers' shotguns going off in his direction. No one knows, and the story seems to end there. Tula May, my grandmother, was lucky, I thought. She got a marriage certificate out of it and a name for her baby. Thirty-seven years later when Clarence pulled a like-father-like-son trick on my mother, she had to use a good deal of creativity to come up with a name for me because his was already taken.

Jack asked about my mother and told me how beautiful she was and that he had always been fond of her. I stifled the urge to say that this was one thing he and his father apparently agreed on.

He told me he had seen her a couple of times on trips back to Cleburne when he was a teenager. Once, he said, she showed him a box full of gold watches and invited him to "pick out one." Then, he said, "Mrs. Conner came in and called her aside and they talked for a while. Then Nita came back in and put the box of watches away. It's too bad, because I had already made my selection."

I told him I remembered all that jewelry and that it had disappeared. He said he suspected that Lonnie came back and got it.

We vowed to get together and agreed that it should be soon. "It's too bad this couldn't have happened when we were younger," he said.

Soon after this conversation, we met at Helen's house. Karen, who has been as interested in our new family as I have, went with me.

I was nervous about meeting Jack. As soon as he saw me he said, "He's a Pollock!" (This meant, I found out later, that I resemble Clarence's mother's side of the family.)

In person, Jack can't disguise his gentleness, which is immediately evident in his ready laugh and the softness of his eyes. They are the eyes of a man who feels everything and shows as little as possible. Reflected in them is the melancholy amiability of a loyal son whose father probably equated tenderness with weakness. His gruffness soon evaporated, though, as did the fearsomeness of his dominant personality. He hugged me easily and without pretense. For the photo sessions, he laid his heavy arm on my shoulder. At other times, he teased me, a prerogative, I've been given to understand, of an older brother. He is sixty-two. He called me "Bud" or "Kiddo."

It is strange and joyous at this time in my life to find that I have a brother and sister and new nieces and nephews. I look at it as a gift and try, finally, to abdicate this comfortable throne of resentment I've occupied all these years. It's true that my father is gone and that I was cheated out of the chance to see him, though he knew about me. Why didn't he let me know? A. B. Dodge said he thought he was my father, yet he didn't beat a trail to my door either. It is hard not to take this personally, but it is self-defeating to continue to brandish these feelings of resentment, bitterness, and regret, to use them to condemn the actions of my mother and these men. Circumstances seemed to have overwhelmed them. These were hard decisions, apparently too hard and complicated for simple country folk to make, and there were few counselors in those days.

What about my feelings of betrayal? Abandonment?

Deprivation? These are just three other words that describe the feelings to which I have always had easy access in my storeroom of emotional appliances. Maybe I won't be trafficking in these convenient excuses any longer. For betrayal, I have tried to substitute understanding; for abandonment, restoration; for deprivation, compensation.

Though these men, for reasons I'll never know, chose to ignore me, there have been men in my life who stayed the course. There was Raymond, who took me into the marriage bargain and eventually became my best friend. Whoever I turn out to be after all this, much of it will have been due to his influence.

Then there was my grandfather, who accepted me without question and saw to my needs without complaint. Until his death on March 16, 1982, he had been my greatest inspiration and teacher. He had caught a cold a month before at Aunt Harriet's funeral and developed a cough. The next day he was in such pain that Lindon carried him to his truck in his arms and drove him to the hospital in Cleburne. My grandfather wanted to go to the Santa Fe Hospital at Temple but knew he was too weak to make the trip.

The night before he died I stayed with him all night. Between injections for pain, his deep-blue eyes would brighten and focus on me momentarily. He hadn't breath enough to speak, but he did move his lips once and, to my everlasting regret, I couldn't understand what he was trying to tell me. I wouldn't have been surprised, though, if it had been something like: "Be sure to cut the water off at the house if it looks like it's going to freeze."

I said, "Daddy, can you hear me?"

He nodded that he could.

I said, "I just wanted you to know that I've loved you. And I want you to know how much I appreciate you and Ann-A taking me in and all the things you did for me. You were the best father anybody could ever have."

He was never a demonstrably affectionate man, but he took my hand and held it for a long time after that.

It hurt to give him up, but he was suffering too much to go on living. He hadn't wanted to live since my grandmother died, sixteen months before, just across the hall from the intensive care unit where he now lay. He had made a great effort to go on without her, but his heart was not in it. He put in his garden, mowed the widow ladies' grass in the neighborhood, took out their trash, rode his bicycle to town to pay their bills. He had his garden ready to plant that year but hadn't gotten it done. "It's no good anymore," he once told me. "I don't care about that old garden anymore, even. Because when Ann-A was here and I would stop at dinnertime and come in the house, she'd be a-settin' there in that rocker and she'd get up and we'd eat a little somethin' and watch the news together. Now, I go into that old house and it's the lonesomest old place in the world. Sometimes I have a notion to just take off walkin' and keep on a-goin'."

I remembered those awful minutes after her death and what I had foolishly said to him: "Daddy, are you all right?"

"I won't never be all right again," he said.

After a while, he went home, got into his bed on the back porch, pulled the quilts over his head and cried for twenty-four hours. When he emerged, he took a bath, shaved, and asked someone to take him to the barbershop. "Are we going to bring her out to the house?" he said. Someone told him this wasn't done anymore.

Earlier, I said that since he was the father of his own sons and of my mother, he couldn't have been my father, too. Maybe, in a way, I was wrong about this. I think he considered himself my father. One thing is certain, to him I owe the fundamental values that have shaped my life. As a teenager, afflicted with the middle-class values learned in school and what was said to be good grammar, I had been ashamed of the way he said "holp" instead of "helped," "clomb" instead of "climbed," "fit" instead of "fought" and, of course, he said "et" for "eaten." It wasn't until I studied Old English in graduate school that I learned these were inflected past tenses of these verbs used by educated writers and scholars in England from the tenth century through Chaucer's times. I also thought that his pronunciation of "hundred" as "hunderd" was another example of his illiteracy. Later, of course, I learned that Tennyson pronounced it this way. He rhymed it with "thundered" in "The Charge of the Light Brigade."

Doltishly, I even said once that he knew nothing about the "finer things in life." Hearing this, my Aunt Sarah said, "No, he had the finer things in life all along, and what the world thinks is the finer things is wrong."

AFTERWORD

On October 18, 1994, at 7:15 A.M., Helen died.

We had seen each other only three times, but we were as comfortable together as if we had known each other all our lives. She answered all my questions honestly and gave me good advice about living. Watching her those last four weeks, I also learned about death with dignity.

I had spent the last weekend with her and had plans to come back the next week and locate an apartment nearby for myself. She wanted me to stay with her, but I thought my being there would be too tiring for her. She had Janet and Barbara, granddaughter Darla, and many other loving and devoted family members who saw after her every need. But I wanted to see her every day and was determined to rent a place nearby.

In one of our late-night talks, I said, "I know people who complain and whine if they're sore from aerobics and have to wear a bandage on their arm and park in a handicap zone if they type too much. Yet you laugh and have a happy disposition in the face of death. Nobody would blame you if you complained. Why don't you?"

"Hon, I would if I thought it do any good," she said.

She told me that she had also gone to Santa Fe Elementary, in the 1920s, and our father had started there in 1908, when it was called East Ward. "He only went to the fourth grade," she said, "but he was a big reader. He read every book Louis L'Amour ever wrote." All three of us had the same first grade teacher, Miss Talullah Douse.

My Grandmother Pollock, she told me, lived only a few blocks from where I grew up on English Street. She lived in the house next door to Mrs. Rogers, the lady who fixed my mother's hair. I used sit on the front porch to wait for my mother just a few feet from where my grandmother lived. My mind reeled.

On the Saturday before Helen died, I drove her all over East Texas, both of us having a high old time. We had the best of two worlds—siblings without the rivalry. She scolded me only once: "Stop calling yourself a bastard," she said. She went on to explain that this was a term she reserved for Republican politicians.

We spent the day looking for a place for me to stay. We went to those great small-town shrines, Dairy Queen and Wal-Mart. She took me to the New London cemetery where her husband's grave was still fresh. It had been only four months since he died, also of cancer. She hadn't yet picked out a monument, she said. She planned to do that soon.

At her funeral the minister told the story of how we had found one another in the last few weeks of her life. I had raised her spirits, he said. I resisted an urge to chuckle at the undertaker's name, Keith Snoozy. I believe Helen would have seen the humor, too.

I sat beside Jack. The night before, he and I had slept in twin beds. It was just like camp, Barbara said. Before the funeral he took me aside and said, "I don't have a necktie. Did you bring an extra one?" I hadn't, but I located one that had belonged to Sid, Helen's late husband. It was one of those clip-on models. He wanted me to help him with getting it on. His collar was too tight, and I had trouble getting it buttoned. With his ersatz fearsome bluster he growled that I had included a section of his skin when I forced the button through the buttonhole. Again, the prerogative of the older brother.

As he was leaving I asked him when he intended to retire. He said he had worked hard all his life and didn't know anything else to do with himself. And he is raising two granddaughters, an obligation that will keep him in the work force for a few more years. But he has a dream— to drive around the country, just himself and Marlene, his wife, maybe see the redwood forest again, this time with no children. Backing out of the driveway, he said, "I don't like writing very much, Bud, but you seem to, so send me a letter now and then."

I talk with Barbara and Janet regularly, and we visit as often as we can, just like any other family. I have been to Alvin, where Jack showed me all the places where they lived, our father's old stomping grounds, like the Top Dog, a saloon that is still standing, and the cemetery where he is buried. I've learned the names of all my new nieces and nephews. I've heard from other relatives and from devoted friends of Helen from around the state. Charles has taught me to hold a rope. He has hopes that I will someday be able to twirl it and throw it in the general direction of a steer without falling off my horse. I got calls from a new aunt in Tolar and from Uncle Bill Booth in Fort Worth. He is Clarence's half brother. He said, "I can tell you all about your daddy for the first thirty years. Your Uncle Dub in Cleburne can tell you the rest."

A few days later Uncle Bill and his wife, Doris, came by for a visit. He is in his eighties but looks twenty years younger. He has a young and attractive wife. They have been married only a few years. He was very interested in my story and eager to tell me what he could about my father. "You look more like Clarence than Jack does," he told me. "You favor the Pollock side of the family, that's mine and Clarence's granddaddy." He said he spent a lot of his early years with Clarence because he was a lot of fun to be with. "But your daddy was one rough customer," he told me. "Nobody in Cleburne ever wanted to tangle with him." He went on to explain that one of my father's occupations was a little dangerous: he worked for the Vaughn boys, bootleggers, supplying moonshine whiskey to honky-tonks in east Cleburne during the Depression.

"What about the police?" I asked, naive as a choir boy.

"Oh, the police wouldn't bother you unless you got behind on your payments," he said. "Except on occasion when Clarence thought they were harassing him too much. He laid one of them out once, and it took eight stitches to close the gash. That cost Clarence a $100 fine."

My father loved his work, apparently, and the whiskey, the gambling, and the girls who went along with it. "He wasn't faithful to Corine, but she put up with it," Uncle Bill said. "There was many a time that she would call me and we'd go looking for him. I knew all his hangouts. We'd eventually find him in one of his honky-tonks and bring him home. He never put up a fight; he'd just come along with us. He was that way," Uncle Bill went on, "but you couldn't help but like him. He was the best-hearted soul you ever saw. There wasn't a thing he wouldn't do for you, if he liked you. But if he didn't, watch out. Even if he didn't know you he'd help you if you were being beat up by two guys. He was always for the underdog. Yessir, your daddy was one tough customer."

He pointed toward a picture of Lindon on the wall and said, "That boy looks a lot like Clarence when he was that age."

He wanted to know what I did for a living. I said I had

been a teacher for twenty-nine years, providing a commodity not nearly so highly sought after or appreciated as the one my father provided.

A few days before Christmas of that year, Jack came and we loaded up his truck and went to my Hill County cabin. I had never been deer hunting before. We built a crackling fire in the stove and talked till midnight. Through the uncurtained windows, I watched the full moon rise over the trees like old Cyclops' eye. I went outside and heard a rustle of leaves—an armadillo came toward me in a shambling, clumsy gait, attracted by my flashlight. A few minutes later a chorus of coyotes erupted suddenly, filling the night with their strange, primordial, sirenlike song. It ceased, after a minute or two, as abruptly as it began. Jack saw it rather as a kind of canine board meeting. "Whatever it was," he said, "they got it settled."

Inexperienced in hunting, I expected to be out there at daybreak, in the ambuscade position. But daylight came, and Jack made no move toward the door. After a pot of coffee and several cigarettes, he was still spinning stories, showing no interest in loading up. Ten o'clock came. Finally, I said, "Shouldn't we have already been out there, in the stalking mode, crouched and ready to blast?"

"Hey, Bud, what you're going to have to learn is there's more to deer hunting than just shooting," he said. That's when I figured out this secret between men: it's a fraternity as old and as sacred as the Dionysian mysteries or the Lion's Club. It isn't just the shooting. It's also the planning, loading the truck with provisions, the roaring fire, the coyotes' song, the beer and beef jerky, breakfast bacon sizzling and spattering on the wood stove the next morning, the hot, cinder-filled coffee, the tall tales spun into the deep of the moonlit night until they are ended, mercifully, only by exhaustion and, most of all, it is the escape from the civilized chaos of freeways and shopping malls.

By noon, though, we were finally out there, armed but posing little threat to the wildlife. We saw one of the coyotes that had performed the night before. It loped slowly toward a stand of trees, stopped, looked back at us over its shoulder, before disappearing into the thicket. We also saw three deer, but they, too, were allowed to move into the woods and disappear without drawing fire. We stalked them, though, and Jack taught me to follow their tracks down the sandy road until they changed direction and jumped the neighbor's fence.

Without his father, or his sons, or friends, to whom he may have felt obliged to demonstrate his skills, with only this bookish brother who had rather study the prey than stalk it, Jack never came close to pulling the trigger. It was almost as if there had been an unspoken pact between us: he wouldn't kill a deer if I wouldn't quote from Thoreau. We would just be ourselves; we were brothers with no baggage of sibling rivalry and no image to uphold. He was right. There is more to hunting than shooting. He had passed up the opportunity to shoot a deer, and I had learned to be more tolerant of hunters.

We visited Uncle Dub Booth at his apartment in Cleburne. At eighty-one, he is only a remnant of skin and bone, deaf but alert, full of fire and wit, and as tightly compacted as a hackberry knot. He literally lives on Ensure laced with bourbon. "The whiskey's the only thing that will cut this phlegm in my head," he said in his metallic voice. "I'm in a helluva damned mess, Jack. I can't hear, my teeth are breaking off at the gums, and I had to quit eating two years ago. It's a damn shame the way they're ripping off the old people. They went up on

Ensure from $16 to $32. I had a scratch on my eyeball, and I went to this lady doctor right here at Kimbro Clinic, and she looked at it and said, 'You've got a scratch on your eyeball,' and charged me $200. It's a damn shame the way they're ripping off the old people."

For our benefit he turned up his hearing aid so loud that I could hear the high-pitched sound it made, like a smoke alarm going off, but he was apparently oblivious to it. "They won't adjust the damn thing," he said, "until I get my ears cleaned out. They say there's fungus growing in there. Same thing with my false teeth. They won't fit but the dentist won't do a damn thing about it. I'm in a helluva damn mess."

He sat in his recliner, his Best Buy cigarettes at hand on an end table covered with a towel. On the other side was a lamp without a shade. To look for photos he wanted to show me, he unscrewed the bulb and replaced it with one the size of a floodlight. When he switched it on, it looked like a nuclear blast went off in the room. When Jack smiled, he said, "Hell, I can't see to read with a hundred watts! I'm in a helluva damn mess, Jack!"

He was thrilled to see us show up together. The stories flowed out of him almost too fast for me to absorb them. "Your father was the best there ever was," he told us. "There wasn't a thing he wouldn't do for you. One day we were heading for the deer lease and I got into a little old fender-bender with this guy that pulled out in front of me. Clarence was following behind me in his truck and saw what happened. The guy was a lot bigger than me and kept saying I did this and I did that to his car and what was I going to do about it. Clarence had pulled over by this time and was listening. When the guy asked me one time too many what I was going to do about it, Clarence said, 'He's not going to do anything about it. The question is, what are you going to do about it?' Well, then, the guy kind of backed off and said he didn't reckon there was all that much damage and he was willing to let it go if I was. And that was the end of it. You better believe it, Clarence was a helluva fellow. In the old days, the police had just as soon not have to mess with Clarence Mann."

"When they came to arrest him," Jack said, matter-of-factly, "they had to have a minimum of four, preferably six."

Uncle Dub walked us to the truck, which was parked beside his Dodge Dakota, complete with camper. "Insurance on it's gone up to over $600 every six months!" he thundered. "It's a damn shame the way they rip off the old people!"

He asked about my mother and wanted her address and phone number. He said he was going to pay her a visit. I told him she was fine.

She is more at peace with herself now. The "old ladies" don't bother her anymore about her past. Now they only say things like they never saw anyone who keeps pictures of the family in her curio cabinet or that her iron bedstead looks like it came out of a farmhouse. She took down the oil painting of the farmhouse Raymond was born in and put it in the closet because the "old ladies" said they wouldn't want anyone to know they were born in such a place. Pretty minor stuff compared to the pain they used to bring her with their comments about her past.

We spend a lot less time together now, which is better for both of us. I've learned many things since Raymond died, not the least of which is that I can't allow myself to feel obligated to make her happy. And I reached a point where I stopped trying to reason with her. I discovered that it made no difference whether she understood that she had flown to Houston or taken a bus. If she lost her purse or the TV clicker or her watch or her beads or her marriage license or her keys, she would just have to find those things herself. I resisted the temptation once, when she asked why I wouldn't help her look for her purse, to say that I was too busy looking for a lost father. But I didn't need to say this. The liberating discovery that I didn't have to concern myself with these never-ending frustrations of hers was satisfying enough.

Her frustration is only momentary. Her joy and anger are momentary, too. Knowing this, I spend my time with her now in a shallow stream of moments that flow like water. How could something so simple be so hard to understand? As my former brother-in-law said to me once when I was confused over a simple loophole used by restaurant owners to sell liquor in a dry area, it was "way over the head of a college professor." It took nearly three years for me to learn this simple fact and to see that I was also trying to make her life perfect by running to her every time she called, behaving as if she were the most important thing in my world.

Looking back, it seems absurd that I did these things. There was no epiphany, no blinding light on the road to Cleburne, just an undramatic recognition of the hold she had on me, a hold I may never understand, except that I apparently have a compulsion toward earning love through some kind of masochistic generosity. My defense was that she is a good person, has a great heart and, most important, she is my mother. She was in trouble and needed me. And, I think she wanted the truth to come out as much as I did. I think she knew her mind was going fast. Among her things in the trunk I discovered this bit

that someone had given her or that she had
where and saved:

ᵉ to say I'm living
That I'm not among the dead;
Though I'm getting more forgetful,
And more mixed up inside my head.

At times I can't remember
While standing on the stair,
If I must go up for something
Or just came down from there.

And before the fridge so often
My mind is filled with doubt:
Have I just put the food away, or
Have I come to take some out?

So, if it's my turn to write you
There's no need in getting sore,
What if I have written
And you think that I'm a bore?

Here I stand beside the mailbox
With a face so very red,
Instead of mailing you my letter—
I've opened it instead!

Unfortunately, neither title nor author was recorded
with this poem.

She lives with minimal complaint, if not contentedly,
in a retirement home again, and I visit her but no longer
in the torturously dutiful way as before. I see more of the
rest of my family now, and my new family. I don't worry
about her because she has supervision, good meals and
housekeeping, dominoes, outings to musicals and the like,

and community with her friends among the other residents.

Visits with her are much more relaxed than before. I know now that putting this distance between us was necessary. Sometimes distance can bring people closer together, though this doesn't seem likely for us. She isn't really of this world anymore but of the world of time past. She is my closest living link to that world, and I value our excursions into distant recollections. But I'm also looking forward to a better life, for all of us, in the world of time present.

CHRONOLOGY

1914 – C. R. Conner marries Annie May James.

1915 – W. L. (Coon) Conner born.

1917 – Howard Conner born; C. R. Conner almost dies from typhoid.

1918 – Uncle Dock, twin brother of Ann-A, dies in World War I; baby Howard Conner dies; Juanita Conner born.

1919 – Wayne Conner born.

1921 – Bernice Conner born.

1937 – Mann family moves to James Street.

1938 – Mann family moves to Alvin; Juanita Conner follows them.

1939 – The author (Tom Dodge) born; Juanita presents baby to A. B. Dodge as his son, takes baby to Cleburne.

1942 – Conner family moves to English Street in Cleburne.

1945 – Author enters Santa Fe Elementary School; Juanita goes to work at Duke & Ayres.

1946 – A. B. Dodge, discharged from army, pays brief visit to Juanita and the author.

1950 – Author enters Cleburne Junior High; W. M., "Grandpa," Conner dies.

1952 – Juanita Conner marries Raymond and moves to Pampa; the author, in trouble at school, follows them to Pampa.

1953 – Author moves back to Cleburne.

1954 – Author moves to Pampa, then back to Cleburne.

1957 – Juanita and Raymond return to Cleburne; the author graduates from high school.

1958 – Author enters military service.

1960 – Author marries Brenda Stinson, goes to work as a fireman for the Texas & Pacific Railway; Lindon Dodge born.

1961 – Author is called back into military.

1962 – Karen Dodge born; the author leaves military service.

1964 – Author graduates from the University of Texas at Arlington, leaves the T&P Railway.

1965 – Author teaches at Mansfield High School.

1967 – Juanita goes to work in the nursery of the First Baptist Church.

1968 – Author receives a Master's Degree from North Texas State University, begins teaching at Blinn College in Brenham; Lowell Dodge born; the author locates A. B. Dodge in Brazoria, Texas.

1970 – Author moves family to Midlothian, begins teaching at Mountain View College; A. B. Dodge killed in automobile crash.

1980 – Annie May Conner (Ann-A) dies.

1982 – C.R. Conner dies; Lindon paralyzed in diving accident.

1991 – Signs of forgetfulness first noticed in Juanita.

1992 – Raymond dies.

1993 – Juanita moves to retirement home, returns to Cleburne six months later.

1994 – Juanita moves to Midlothian in March, returns to retirement home in October; the author retires from teaching, locates the Mann family; Helen Mann Hollingsworth dies two months after the author first meets her.

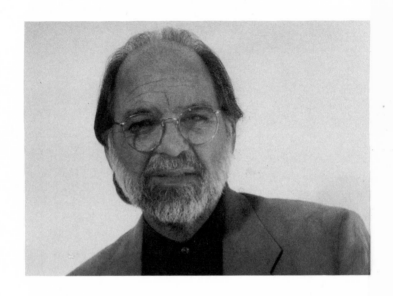

THE AUTHOR

Born in Houston and raised in the small railroad town of Cleburne, Texas, Tom Dodge worked for the Texas & Pacific Railway before going on to teach English at Mansfield High School, Blinn College, and Mountain View College. Today, he is a writer and commentator for Station KERA (National Public Radio) in Dallas. He makes his home in Midlothian, Texas.

He is the author of *A Literature of Sports* (1980) and *A Generation of Leaves* (1977), a translation of Greek Lyrics.